How to Succeed at the Medical Interview

Chris Smith MRCP
GP Registrar
Wessex Deanery
Hampshire

Darryl Meeking MRCP
Consultant Endocrinologist
Honorary Clinical Lecturer
University of Southampton
Honorary Senior Lecturer
University of Portsmouth
Portsmouth

Blackwell
Publishing

BMJ|Books

Blackwell Publishing, Inc., 350 Main Street, Malden, Massachusetts 02148-5020, USA
Blackwell Publishing Ltd, 9600 Garsington Road, Oxford OX4 2DQ, UK
Blackwell Publishing Asia Pty Ltd, 550 Swanston Street, Carlton, Victoria 3053, Australia

First published 2008
3   2009

Library of Congress Cataloging-in-Publication Data
Smith, Chris, 1976–
    How to succeed at the medical interview / Chris Smith, Darryl Meeking.
        p. ; cm.
    Includes index.
    ISBN 978-1-4051-6729-1 (alk. paper)
    1. Medicine–Vocational guidance–Great Britain.   2.
Physicians–Employment–Great Britain.   3. Employment interviewing–Great Britain.   I. Meeking,
Darryl.   II. Title.
    [DNLM: 1. Interviews–Great Britain.   2. Job Application–Great Britain.   3. Physicians–Great
Britain.   W 21 S644h 2008]

    R690.S5443 2008
    610.69–dc22

                                                                                    2007043482

ISBN: 978-1-4051-6729-1

A catalogue record for this title is available from the British Library

Set in 9.5 on 12 pt Minion by SNP Best-set Typesetter Ltd., Hong Kong
Printed and bound in Singapore by COS Printers Pte Ltd

Commissioning Editor: Mary Banks
Development Editor: Simone Dudziak
Production Controller: Rachel Edwards

For further information on Blackwell Publishing, visit our website:
http://www.blackwellpublishing.com

The publisher's policy is to use permanent paper from mills that operate a sustainable forestry policy, and
which has been manufactured from pulp processed using acid-free and elementary chlorine-free practices.
Furthermore, the publisher ensures that the text paper and cover board used have met acceptable
environmental accreditation standards.

Contents

Foreword

Selection into a medical career post has never been under more scrutiny. Chris Smith and Darryl Meeking have offered a very practical guide to success at the medical interview. Their central tenet is that preparation, preparation, preparation should be the applicant's mantra. I am sure this is correct, and their book gives a myriad of ways to improve your performance at various selection methods.

The authors give sound advice on everything and remind applicants that honesty and integrity are key attributes of a doctor, and to resist any temptation to overembellish. The guide is full of examples of where things have gone slightly wrong in these and other areas from the viewpoints of the applicant and the selector.

It is traditional to wish candidates good luck before a selection process. Following Smith and Meeking's advice may not minimise the amount of good fortune you will need to be successful, but you can be confident that you could not have prepared more thoroughly. Good luck!

Professor Frank Smith
Director of Postgraduate GP Education
Wessex Deanery
NHS Education South Central

Acknowledgements

We are very grateful to our friends and colleagues who have helped us and shared their interview experiences with us, in particular Dr Penny Wilson, Dr John-Paul Smith, Dr Adam Kirk, Dr Helen Pedgrift, Dr Howard Smith and Dr Sarah Gorman.

We would especially like to thank Dr Tom Walton and Dr Sameer Trikha for checking the text and for their incredibly helpful comments.

Finally, our thanks go to our friends and families for all of their support.

Introduction

In the UK, doctors generally prepare poorly for the medical interview. Surprisingly, little or no thought is given to preparation, yet a successful medical career is entirely dependent upon results at interview.

Doctors often invest many months, thousands of pounds and vast amounts of energy into stressful medical examinations that carry with them no guarantee of a chosen career path. Much less effort is spent in preparing for the medical interview, although the failure rate for the most competitive interviews is far higher than that of postgraduate exams.

The interview is a highly competitive process that may favour certain personality types, but the key to success lies in thorough preparation. The evidence for this is strong:

An interviewer's perspective

I have interviewed many hundreds of doctors, all differing in personality and competency and with a variety of strengths and weaknesses. Following selection I have worked with many of these doctors and I have discovered the interview process to be, at best, variable in its ability to detect and appoint the best individuals.

Do not be deceived into thinking that the best doctors succeed at interview and the worst fail. I have seen nervous, weak and uncertain doctors shine immeasurably in the face of a barrage of hostile questioning at interview. Conversely, I have seen warm, confident and knowledgeable doctors disintegrate into quivering wrecks when asked a straightforward question by a polite, smiling interviewer.

Continued

How to Succeed at the Medical Interview By C. Smith and D. Meeking. 2008 by Blackwell Publishing, ISBN: 978-1-4051-6729-1.

Continued

> I have witnessed some individuals at every training grade from Medical student to Consultant, and have interviewed them at different stages during their career.
>
> I have seen one hopelessly unprepared doctor perform dismally at interview, giving the impression to the panel that she was strange, distant and cold. Following a feedback telephone conversation an hour later that same doctor emerged as warm, engaging and confident. One year later, she was successful at interview for the same training programme after a more thorough programme of preparation.
>
> *I have therefore become convinced that it is good preparation, and not a person's ability or personality that is the key to success at the medical interview.*

Doctors are likely to undergo several interviews of different types during their career. To our knowledge, this is the first book produced that will enable you to prepare thoroughly for most, if not all, forms of medical interview. This book is aimed primarily at postgraduate interviews, although there are elements that may be of use to those preparing for Medical School entrance interviews.

What is an interview?

Important note!

For the purpose of this book, the term 'Interview' is used to encompass any form of selection for a post where you are being assessed in person. In recent years, newer models for selecting candidates have emerged, complementing or even replacing the traditional structured interview. For instance, you may be invited to attend an assessment day, or another re-branded form of selection, but for simplicity we will use the term 'Interview' throughout this book.

How to use this book

We will stress repeatedly that preparation is the key to success in the medical interview. With this in mind, it is essential that you discover the format of the selection process you will be undertaking so that you can use this book as effective preparation.

- Chapter 1 will describe the different types of medical interview
- Chapter 2 will give important information about how to prepare for your interview

- Chapter 3 will help you to optimise your performance at all types of interview
- Chapter 4 will provide you with information about questions that are commonly asked at interview and how to answer them
- Chapter 5 will give you information about knowledge-based questions that are currently asked at interview
- Chapter 6 provides you with likely questions that test your generic skills and how you should answer them
- Chapter 7 aims to help you prepare for the competency-based assessments and tasks now frequently used as part of the interview process.

Although the theme of interview questions may be similar for interviews at all levels, some questions are more likely to be asked at some grades and types of medical interview than for others. You should focus your attention on those aspects most relevant for your career stage and career choice. We endeavour to highlight these differences wherever possible.

Good luck!

Chapter 1 **The medical interview**

> The aims of this chapter are to give an overview of:
> - The application process prior to the interview
> - The aims of the medical interview
> - The different types of medical interview
> - The make-up and role of the different members of the interview panel
> - The types of questions asked at the medical interview
> - How candidates are selected

1.1 The application process

Although the main focus of this book is on the interview stage, it is important to cover the process that precedes the interview. This will vary according to the post for which you are applying.

The Modernising Medical Careers (MMC) process has led to the development of Foundation programme (F1 and F2) and Specialist Training programmes for each specialty (ST1, ST2, ST3, etc.).

For the majority of Foundation posts, candidates are matched and interviews are not carried out. However, for Foundation posts that remain vacant, a short-listing and interview process is still used to select appropriate candidates.

For those who are applying for Specialist Training (ST) or General Practice (GP) training, the short-listing is undertaken by Deanery-based selection panels. Selection consists of a structured interview process. You are advised to check the MMC website for updated information that relates to your chosen specialty (see later).

Structured application forms may be preferred as the basis for short-listing and interviewing candidates rather than the traditional curriculum vitae (CV).

How to Succeed at the Medical Interview By C. Smith and D. Meeking. 2008 by Blackwell Publishing, ISBN: 978-1-4051-6729-1.

However, there are many situations in which CVs are likely to be requested. The most likely posts that CVs will be required for are:

- Vacant Foundation posts
- Trust doctor posts
- Senior medical posts.

For GP training there are three stages that candidates need to undergo in order to get selected:

- Stage 1: an application form (this may be online), the purpose of which is to check the eligibility of the candidate
- Stage 2: a written assessment under exam conditions. This could involve an MCQ (multiple choice questions) exam or essay questions that test generic skills
- Stage 3: an interview.

How are candidates short-listed for ST and GP training posts?

Each post comes with a Person Specification and consists of entry criteria (minimum standards) and selection criteria. The entry criteria allow non-medical staff to screen candidates prior to short-listing. Those who are short-listing decide who should be interviewed according to the selection criteria. There will usually be an agreed subset of *main* selection criteria:

Entry criteria
- Qualifications
- Eligibility
- Career progression
- Fitness to practise
- Health
- Language skills
- A 'complete application'

Selection criteria
- Clinical skills
- Personal skills
- Commitment to specialty
- Probity
- Academic and research achievements

It is vital that you read through the Person Specification criteria for the post that you are applying for in detail.

Here is an example of requirements for an ST1 post in General Medicine:

Entry criteria for ST1 in General Medicine (mostly obtained from the application form)

Qualifications
- Appropriate medical qualification, e.g. MBBS

Eligibility
- Eligible for GMC registration
- Evidence of achievement of Foundation competencies in line with GMC standards/good medical practice including:

Good clinical care
- Maintaining good medical practice
- Good relationships/communication with patients
- Good working relationships with colleagues
- Good teaching and training
- Professionalism/probity
- Delivery of good acute clinical care
- Eligibility to work in the UK

Fitness to practise
- Up to date and fit to practise safely

Language skills
- Capable of effective communication with patients/colleagues (medical training in English or appropriate IELTS scores)
- Health
- Meets professional health requirements
- Career progression
- Can provide complete employment history details
- Less than 12 months' experience at SHO level (not foundation)

Selection criteria for ST1 post in General Medicine (from application form and subsequently from interview and references)

Clinical skills
- Appropriate knowledge base and ability to apply clinical judgement

Personal skills
- Communication: adapting language appropriate to situation
- Problem solving/decision making: using logic and thought to solve and decide
- Managing others/teamwork: working effectively with others
- Sensitivity/empathy: taking in others' perspectives and treating others with understanding

Continued

Continued

- Organisation/planning: managing and prioritising time and situations effectively
- Vigilance/situational awareness: monitoring and anticipating issues
- Coping with pressure: operating under pressure, initiative and resilience

Probity
- Professional integrity: takes responsibility and respects all others

Commitment to specialty
- Other activities and achievements relevant to medicine

Academic/research skills
- Demonstrates understanding of audit and research
- Evidence of academic/research achievements (desirable)
- Participation in audit (desirable)
- Experience and interest in teaching (desirable)

Useful websites

- National GP recruitment: www.gprecruitment.org
- Modernising Medical Careers: www.mmc.nhs.uk

1.2 The aims of the medical interview

Why does the medical interview exist?

Historically, across all spectra of business and industry, the interview has been used to select applicants for posts, with candidates usually having been short-listed on the basis of an application form or CV.

The interview gives employers the opportunity to meet potential employees face to face and decide if they wish to employ that person. It provides an opportunity to test applicants' competencies and motivation in a structured environment, thereby attempting to provide a level playing field on which the best applicants can shine.

Medical interviews are no different in this respect, and the aim is to select the best candidate for the vacant post.

Does everything hinge on the medical interview?

There may be factors other than performance at interview that impact on whether a candidate is successful. Some candidates will have an advantage based upon their past experience and performance, including their responses to questions on the application form. As part of some selection processes (such as GP) there is a written assessment under exam conditions. A good perform-ance, or additional qualifications or experience, may add to the overall strength of a candidate's application.

It is also possible that candidates will have gained an advantage prior to interview through previous contact with members of the panel. Occasionally an interviewer has witnessed a candidate's performance first-hand in the work-place. In other instances, a trusted colleague may have recommended a candi-date to a panel member. Sometimes candidates have made the effort to meet with panel members for the first time prior to interview, but this is frequently not possible.

However, do not fall into the trap of thinking that the outcome of an inter-view is predetermined. This is rarely the case, and is frequently used by unsuc-cessful applicants as an easy excuse to explain their failure.

There can be no doubt that it is the most crucial component of candidate selection. The interview process, in whatever shape or form it takes, is labour-intensive for those who are organising and running it. Applicants who have made it to that stage will be of similar calibre, and an interview performance may be the only way to distinguish between them.

What does the interviewer expect?

Much is made of the personal biases of people who sit on interview panels, and naturally there may be individual preferences according to personalities and styles. You may be surprised to know that there is usually broad agree-ment amongst interview panel members when it comes to selection. In other words, the best candidate is usually obvious. Your aim should be to convince the panel that you are the best candidate. The key to achieving this is good preparation!

Remember (this might sound obvious), each member of the interview panel usually wants to select the best candidate at interview.

1.3 Types of medical interview

For many years the format of the medical interview has been similar for all grades of doctor, except that with increasing seniority longer interviews and larger interview panels could be expected.

Recently, however, in many cases the traditional medical interview has been supplemented or replaced with other mechanisms for selecting candidates. These may include competency-based tasks.

A loose distinction can be made between the older style 'traditional medical interview' and newer interviews that incorporate competency-based tasks.

We encourage you not to think of these as mutually exclusive, as medical interviews frequently incorporate elements of both.

In general, interviews are carried out in an educational setting based within a Hospital, General Practice or Deanery.

1.4 The traditional medical interview

This is the type of interview that many senior doctors will be familiar with. The interview typically involves a panel of interviewers asking a series of questions, with all candidates being asked similar questions.

Interviews may last anything from 15 minutes to 1 hour. Shorter interviews generally occur with smaller interview panels.

For ST posts, the national recommendation is that a minimum of 30-minute interview slots are allocated to applicants who have been successfully short-listed. Interviews for Consultant posts typically last for 1 hour.

1.5 Competency-based assessments

The idea of using different selection tools, other than the traditional interview, to select doctors is relatively new. It is, however, a commonly used selection method for recruiting in the business world, and we discuss these tasks at length in Chapter 7.

Competency-based assessments have a well-established role in the selection of GP trainees and have now been implemented in most ST interviews.

Assessments are designed to test various competencies, with an emphasis on generic skills rather than the candidate's clinical knowledge or past experience. Examples of exercises include:
- Patient simulation exercises
- Prioritisation exercises
- Group tasks
- Making a presentation
- Written exercises
- Tests of medical knowledge.

How is a competency-based interview day structured?
Typically, a Postgraduate Educational Centre is the location for a competency-based interview. Approximately 30–40 candidates are assessed during the day. Candidates will normally have three or four assessments, each lasting 30 minutes. Candidates should expect to spend at least half a day at the centre. A typical timetable for a competency-based interview is as follows:

Structure of a GP competency-based interview

Registration: 16.30 to 16.55
Location: Reception area

Written exercise: 17.00 to 17.30
Location: Room 1

Patient simulation: 17.30 to 18.00
Location: Room 2

Group exercise: 18.00 to 18.30
Location: Room 3

Admin: 18.45 to 18.50
Location: Reception area

Complete forms: 18.50 onwards — then free to leave

1.6 The interview panel

For ST posts there are national recommendations for England, Wales and Northern Ireland that determine who should be present on interview panels. You can expect the following people:

• Lay chairperson
• Regional College adviser or deputy
• Postgraduate Dean or deputy
• Programme Director or chair of Specialty Training Committee
• 2–4 Consultants from training locations
• A Trust Senior Manager
• University representative (for academic posts).

Frequently, however, Deanery-based interviews may consist of as few as two Consultants and a lay member.

If the interview consists of a number of stations, there are usually two interviewers allocated to each station.

The interview panel for stand-alone or trust-grade posts typically consists of a number of consultants (any number between 1 and 10) and a representative from Medical Personnel who takes no part in the decision-making process. When a post is relevant to just one department, it is not unusual to find just two interviewers.

Interviews at Consultant level will include a Senior Manager (typically the Chief Executive or Medical Director), and a representative from the appropriate Royal College and from the Deanery.

In academic institutions there may be a University representative present for interviews for ST level and above. This is usually an academic clinician at a Consultant-equivalent grade.

Although Medical Personnel departments and Deaneries will not usually give out the details of those involved in the short-listing process, it should be possible to discover in advance who will make up the panel.

Those individuals involved in the short-listing process will usually make up part or all of the interview panel.

1.7 Questions asked at the medical interview

How are interview questions decided?

Fortunately, with the traditional interview, the types of questions that you are likely to be asked are fairly predictable. Naturally, for senior medical posts, questions may be more difficult, but the preparation should be similar for whichever post you are applying for.

Typically, the format of the traditional medical interview will be as follows:

- Questions about your CV and medical career to date
- Questions about your portfolio
- Questions that test your motivation. Why this job? Why this area? Why should we choose you?
- Questions about audit and/or research
- Questions about NHS (e.g. MMC) and management topics
- Questions about medicine (e.g. recent articles read/recent advances/medical knowledge)
- Questions that test your generic skills
- Questions about your interests outside of medicine
- An opportunity for you to ask questions.

At least one interviewer will choose to run through the candidate's experience to date, and this is often the opening enquiry. This question gives the candidate an opportunity to provide a quick summary of their medical career and experience to date whilst enabling them to relax ahead of potentially more difficult questions.

This will be followed by questions from other interviewers that will focus on all other aspects of their CV, their motivation, their understanding of health policy, knowledge of relevant literature, education and ethical issues.

At interview, each panel member will decide in advance which questions they are going to ask. Interviewers may have their personal favourite questions that they consider to be 'discriminatory'. It is considered good interview practice for the same questions to be asked of each candidate (although this is rarely adhered to rigidly).

For this reason, you may wish to enquire gently of departing candidates the nature of questions they received. However, be wary of information received from those you don't know or trust.

Our advice is that you should not tell other candidates the questions that you have been asked.

The following statements regarding interview questions are likely to be true:
- Questions will be based on the relevant person specification
- Questions will be consistent across interviewers and for all candidates
- Questions will be scored according to a scoring framework that links to the Person Specification.

Although minimum standards for training posts have been agreed nationally, the interview format is decided by the local Deanery and the individual specialty, so that there will be significant variation between interview centres.

All of these topics and other commonly asked questions are covered in detail in the rest of this book.

1.8 Candidate selection at interview

During an interview, each member of the panel will adjudicate and score the candidate. Each panel member is asked to score an individual according to a number of characteristics that are considered important for the post.

Each member of the interview panel plays an equal part in adjudicating, with the exception of the Medical Personnel officer, those simply sitting in for interview experience and sometimes the chairman. A simple scoring form looks something like this:

Name	Experience (score 1–5)	Qualifications (score 1–5)	Other factors (score 1–5)	Overall impression (score 1–5)	Comments	Rating (score 1–5)

With this scoring system, there is plenty of scope for subjective assessment on behalf of the interviewer. Increasingly, more detailed forms are being developed, based upon essential and desirable criteria.

Below is an example interview question about coping with stress for an ST1 training post in General Medicine. After the question, you will note a number of positive and negative indicators that help to guide the interviewers. A scoring scale accompanies these indicators. This helps provide an assessment of candidates that is based upon objective measurements.

'Describe a time when pressure at work has led to you feeling angry'

Probes: What was the cause?
         What did you do?
         What was the outcome?

Indicators

Positive indicators	Negative indicators
• Remained calm	• Defensive or uncompromising
• Aware of wider situation	• Only dealt with immediate needs
• Knows when to seek help	• Used inappropriate coping strategies
• Responds quickly and decisively	• Hesitant and unsure
• Uses strategies to deal with stress	• Dealt with situation alone
• Recognises own limitations	

Scoring scale

0	No evidence	No evidence reported
1	Poor	Little evidence of positive indicators
		Mostly negative indicators, many decisive
2	Areas for concern	Limited number of positive indicators
		Many negative indicators, one or more decisive
3	Satisfactory	Satisfactory display of positive indicators
		Some negative indicators but none decisive
4	Good to excellent	Strong display of positive indicators
		Few negative indicators and all minor

With interviews that involve a number of stations, trained assessors evaluate and score candidates' performance during each exercise. Information is then summated for each candidate in separate files. After the final exercise, an assessor studies each file. The assessor should have had no earlier involvement with that candidate and provides an independent evaluation of every doctor's performance.

Assessors then discuss performance across all exercises, and selection decisions are made. An independent facilitator oversees this process and asks assessors to provide evidence for their evaluations, in order to increase objectivity and fairness. Decisions are based on the evidence observed according to objective parameters similar to those outlined in the above example. The objective is to avoid decisions based upon 'gut feeling' or unsubstantiated judgements.

After all of the interviews have been completed, the final rating scores are added up and the posts are offered in order according to which candidate ranks most highly. If there is a choice of posts, then the candidate ranking most highly gets first choice.

Important! All interview selection processes should not discriminate against those candidates who are willing to accept some posts but not others.

Generally, this principle is adhered to and it is in your best interests to be honest about which posts you are interested in and which you are not.

How do candidates find out if they are successful?
With Consultant and stand-alone posts, candidates are likely to be told on the day of the interview if they have been successful. This may take the form of the successful candidates being invited back to the interview room, or being telephoned. Formal confirmation may then follow in the post.

Selection for ST programmes can be fairly time consuming. Candidates may have to wait for several somewhat anxious days before they discover whether they have been successful, and will be informed by telephone or e-mail.

Before a final decision is made, there is a review of the candidates' references. A more formal offer is then usually sent by post within a few days. Unsuccessful candidates should be given the opportunity for face-to-face or telephone feedback.

What does an interview process feel like?
Some of you may not have been interviewed before. We thought it would be helpful to recall the experience of one interview candidate.

A candidate's ST1 interview experience

My ST1 Ophthalmology interview consisted of two interview panels each interviewing for 15 minutes, although speaking to friends going through the same process, this varied between Deaneries. Some Deaneries elected to stick to a one-panel 30-minute interview. As a rule, interview time was 30 minutes as a minimum, and included examination of candidates' portfolios. The emphasis was placed upon generic medical skills and aspects of good medical practice. Assessment focused upon the Person Specifications. The following areas were included:
- Commitment to the specialty
- Practical skills (specialty specific)
- Teamwork and communication skills

Continued

Continued

- Management skills
- Decision-making skills
- Critical appraisal skills
- Presentation skills.

One member of the panel was assigned to examining and then marking my portfolio. The first interview station included a 'history taking' type OSCE, similar to Medical School Finals, lasting approximately 6–7 minutes. This tested a range of skills such as acquiring necessary information using a series of open and closed questions, addressing expectations, beliefs and concerns, etc. It appeared that the panel had a 'mark sheet' on which points were allocated.

Part two of the interview involved a practical assessment. Candidates were either asked to examine fundi, using a direct ophthalmoscope, or use microsurgical instruments to demonstrate suturing. In other Deaneries, panels assessed stereoscopic and binocular vision.

Prior to the second interview station, I had been given a scientific paper to read for 20 minutes. I was immediately questioned on the strengths and weaknesses of the paper, with reference to the study methodology, and asked what I would change in the scientific method. The panel were using two or three different scientific journals to minimise candidates discussing the papers. In other Deaneries, candidates were asked to appraise and then present a paper using Microsoft PowerPoint. This indirectly assessed their IT skills.

Other interview questions I was asked included:

- 'As a member of a clinical trial, you have suspicions that a treatment is harming patients. What would you do and why?'
- 'Tell us about a time when you made a mistake. What did you do? What happened?'
- 'Tell me about a time when you were involved in clinical audit'
- 'You come into work and a colleague is drunk, what would you do?'
- 'What is consent? How would you consent a patient? Do you think you should consent a patient for a procedure?'

The interviews generally followed a structured format so appearing to maximise objectivity, and were strictly run to time. In my experience, there was generally little opportunity to ask questions at the end. I noticed immediate reactions when certain words or phrases such as 'communication' or 'patient safety' were mentioned, giving the implication of indicators in the answers determining a score. As each question was predefined, it was more difficult to establish a rapport with the panel members.

It was evident from the interviews that panels were keen to assess candidates across a range of skills, as outlined in the Person Specifications.

1.9 Summary

- Although the format of the medical interview may vary, interview questions will broadly fall into predictable categories
- The competency-based assessment focuses on testing a candidate's generic skills and competencies for the post, and may or may not include a structured interview
- Interviewers try, as much as possible, to be objective when scoring, and selecting successful candidates
- Effective preparation is the key to success.

Chapter 2 **Preparing for the interview**

2.1 Introduction

The aim of this chapter is to give you a framework that will help you prepare thoroughly for the medical interview.

If your interview is tomorrow, then you should focus on the common questions section in this book (Chapter 4). If you have more time, then you should find out about the structure of your interview in detail and then work through this book chapter by chapter. You can omit the few sections that are not relevant to the interview process that you will be undergoing.

Thorough preparation prior to interview will reduce the nerves you experience on the day!

2.2 Know yourself

It is worth spending some time getting to know yourself before an interview. If you were sitting in your living room with your best friend, would you be able to provide succinct answers to these questions, without thinking about them first?
- 'Tell me about yourself'
- 'What annoys you?'
- 'What are your strengths and weaknesses?'

If, with no audience, it takes you 20 minutes of soul searching to answer these questions, then you will struggle to answer questions about yourself in the pressurised situation of an interview within 2 minutes and with six people staring at you!

The best candidates are able to provide concise, personal answers. Some people find it quite easy to talk about their character traits, probably because

How to Succeed at the Medical Interview By C. Smith and D. Meeking. 2008 by Blackwell Publishing, ISBN: 978-1-4051-6729-1.

they do so in day-to-day conversation, and the medical interview is essentially a formal discussion. If you are not one of these people, then you will need to practise.

The more thinking you do before your interview, the less thinking you will need to do on the day. The following chapters will look at these sorts of questions in more detail. By the time you have finished reading this book, you should know yourself much better.

Here are some more examples of questions that require you to understand yourself:
- 'Describe your character'
- 'Think of three adjectives that describe you'
- 'What are you good at and why?'

2.3. Perfecting your curriculum vitae/application form

Is this the end of the road for the CV?

For the purposes of this section we will sometimes use the term 'CV' to encompass CV and application form.

CVs may not be required when applying for medical training posts in the UK, although an up-to-date CV should form part of a doctor's Learning Portfolio which should be brought along to the interview.

A CV is usually required for Consultant and GP posts, as well as for Hospital posts that don't fall under the umbrella of Specialist Training.

How to ensure that you get short-listed

The key to being successfully short-listed for an interview lies in the written information that you provide. It is rarely possible either to know or to be able to influence Consultants who are carrying out the short-listing process. Medical Personnel departments rarely reveal this information.

If you are lucky enough to discover who is short-listing, it might be possible for a referee or a supportive Consultant to influence this process through direct contact with that individual, although this is frowned upon. However, it is not advisable to contact Consultants directly yourself unless you are already on good terms with them and are certain that this would not be perceived negatively.

How to get your CV right

The fundamentals of a good CV are that it should be clear, grammatically precise and set out in the correct order so that the short-listing process is made easier. Many a CV has been rejected without turning the first page. The following simple measures will help your CV stand out from the crowd:

- Use brilliant white or cream paper
- For binding, consider gold-effect clasps or clips (through the paper)
- Send the correct number of CVs asked for
- Allow plenty of time for postage and use registered mail
- For packaging use a Jiffy (or similar) padded bag with cardboard backing to prevent CVs bending in transit.

Your CV should be set out in an attractive way that draws the reader's attention to your strengths. An example of a well-structured CV is given below:

Example CV structure

- Personal details
- Current employment
- Education
- Qualifications
- Awards
- Past employment
- Clinical experience
- Research/audit/publications
- Presentations/teaching
- Management/administrative experience
- Courses/meetings attended
- Hobbies/interests
- References

CV writing services on the web

- www.medicalcvs.com
- www.medical-interviews.co.uk
- www.apply2medicine.co.uk

If you are applying for a post that uses a standardised application form with known assessment criteria, it is essential to obtain this information in advance of applying. You should ensure that you fulfil all of the essential criteria and as many of the desirable criteria as possible. If you cannot meet these criteria you should work towards gaining the experience and qualifications that are required for the post that you are applying for.

Assume that the interview panel have not read your CV!

A popular post will attract many applications.

When you give your answers, do not assume that the interviewers have any prior knowledge of the contents of your CV. It is up to you to draw their attention to your exam successes, audits, research, etc. At interview you may be able to highlight areas of your CV, but you will primarily be selling yourself through your answers to interview questions.

Know your CV inside out!

Everyone on the interview panel should have a copy of your CV or application form in front of them. Many of the interview questions will be based upon this information. You should be prepared for questions about anything that appears within it. This could include an audit you participated in 10 years ago, or, if you have stated an interest in reading, a summary of the book you last read. Therefore, familiarise yourself with your audits and research, and be prepared to talk in detail about every line on your CV.

It is very embarrassing to be asked questions about your CV that you cannot answer. You should therefore remove items that you are no longer familiar with, or that are damaging or irrelevant.

It is particularly dangerous to include facts in your CV or application form that are untrue and can be exposed as such during the interview. It has become increasingly common for any publication lists you produce to be verified prior to interview.

Occasionally inaccuracies can be cruelly exposed at a much later date:

One candidate's tale

I remember many years ago attending an interview with a CV in which I stated a clear interest in sailing. In truth, I had sailed once before but I felt that I should incorporate something other than drinking beer and watching football in my hobbies section. I was relieved that no questions were asked about this during the interview. Unfortunately, 2 months later my Consultant lost his crew and, based upon the CV he had seen at interview, he insisted that I sail with him in a local regatta. I had to confess that I couldn't sail and I'm not sure he trusted me again.

2.4 Your portfolio

It is likely that one of your interviewers will be tasked with looking through and asking about your portfolio. The portfolio of some candidates can be so poor as to penalise them heavily, leaving no possibility of success at interview. It should be made clear to you in advance of your interview whether you need to bring along your portfolio. The exact composition of a Learning Portfolio will vary between different grades of doctor, but typically includes the following:

- An opportunity for self-evaluation
- Discussions with educational supervisor
- A Personal Development Plan
- An educational agreement
- Evidence of reflective learning
- Evidence and assessment of competence
- An up-to-date CV
- Examples of audits, presentations, and certificates of achievement such as ALS.

A well-presented portfolio can earn you useful bonus marks at interview.

If you have positive feedback from colleagues, patients or relatives, this should be highlighted in your portfolio. However, it is important that you should not incorporate confidential patient details.

Further information about portfolios on the web

- www.foundationprogramme.nhs.uk
- www.eportfolio.rcgp.org.uk

2.5 Researching the post

You should have a clear understanding of the post you are applying for prior to being interviewed. As a general rule, you should not apply for a job that you don't want. You should not usually get to the interview stage only to turn it down if you are offered the post. If there are different posts available, or if the post you are offered is not quite the one that you had applied for and you are not sure that you want to accept the post, then you should request a short delay. In this situation, it is reasonable to request 24 hours to ensure that you make the correct decision.

For Consultant posts, you will need to know exactly how many sessions a week you will be working. You will also need to know your clinical, teaching, managerial and administrative responsibilities. For GP posts, you will need to know whether the post is salaried or a partnership, and have a detailed understanding of the financial arrangements for the practice.

For more junior medical positions, you should aim to have a good knowledge of your chosen job specification and location.

Location, location, location!

National or regional application processes for training posts mean that visiting individual hospitals with the aim of getting to meet individual Consultants is of less value than it once was.

It is, however, worth visiting the hub hospital of the rotation that you are applying for.

However, as a minimum, you will state a preference for a region or Deanery as part of your application. With this in mind, familiarise yourself with the Deanery website, and try to crystallise in your mind your reasons for wanting to work in that particular area.

If you are applying for a post at a particular Hospital or General Practice, and you are not an internal candidate, it is definitely still worth arranging an informal visit prior to your interview.

Arranging a visit prior to your interview

Take the opportunity to look at the Hospital or General Practice website. What is the Trust strategy? For example, is the Hospital applying for Foundation status? Can you find a recent report from the Healthcare Commission?

Make arrangements to visit at a convenient time. Try to find out who will be on the interview panel. If allowed, you should aim to meet up with at least one member of the interview panel. In order to do this you should establish a good rapport with the appropriate secretary. The other advantage of knowing who is on the interview panel is that there may be an opportunity for one of your colleagues to put in a good word for you.

If you are applying for a more junior post, try to meet up with the Consultant for whom you would be working if you were successful. You should also make contact with the doctor who is currently in the post that you are applying for.

When visiting, take copies of your CV with you to distribute to senior doctors. You should take the opportunity to ask questions about:

- Teaching and training
- Postgraduate exam pass rates
- Out-of-hours commitments
- What the job is really like!
- What qualities they are looking for in applicants.

Remember that those you are visiting may be busy, so be respectful and don't take up too much of anyone's time. Be presentable and enthusiastic.

Remember that carrying out thorough research of the post for which you are applying will help to decide if the post is right for you and avoid the potential embarrassment of accepting a post and then having to turn it down at a later stage.

2.6 Researching your specialty

A good knowledge of your specialty is expected, and is particularly important for potential trainees hoping to embark on run-through training. The same applies for doctors wishing to change career path, for example from Hospital medicine to General Practice.

Asking others

Take the opportunity in appraisal sessions to discuss your strengths and weaknesses. Discuss your future plans. Consider obtaining formal career advice if you are not sure. Your local Deanery should be able to provide you with specialist careers advice. Making the wrong decisions at an early stage in your career can prove to be costly later on. Your personality and strengths may be more suited to a career in Histopathology than Orthopaedic surgery. It is worth seeking the honest opinions of those who know you and using that information to guide your career decisions.

Reading

There is a wealth of information available about different medical specialties. Make use of books, journals and the internet to find out more about your chosen specialty. At the very least you should know the answers to these questions:
- What is the structure of the training programme?
- What are the 'essential' and 'desirable' criteria required for you to enter the training programme?
- Where will the specialty be in 10 years' time? Is this compatible with where you see yourself in 10 years' time?
- What opportunities are there for research?
- What are the latest developments within the specialty?
- What opportunities are there for sub-specialising?
- What NICE (National Institute for Health and Clinical Excellence) guidelines and National Service Frameworks (NSFs) relate to that specialty?

Gaining experience

Will your chosen specialty be right for you? Specialty experience obtained as part of a Foundation programme is likely to be very different from being involved at Consultant level. For example, as a F2 doing Cardiology you are most likely to spend most of your time on the wards seeing acute in-patient Cardiology. You are not likely to have much exposure to out-patient clinics, or the 'cath lab'. If you are enthusiastic about a specialty and are considering it as a long-term career, make sure you have had exposure to all aspects of the specialty.

If you want to be a GP but didn't have a GP block in your Foundation programme, make sure you arrange to 'sit in' with a GP in your own time.

Think about what you enjoyed at Medical School, but also make sure you have had some exposure at postgraduate level. As well as helping you make the right choice for you, developing 'personal reasons' for entering a specialty will pay dividends at your interview.

Remember that the majority of your career will be spent at the highest level (as a Consultant or GP). Therefore, your decisions should focus on this end-point, and not the comparatively few years spent in training

2.7 Preparing for the questions

You may have a wealth of knowledge and experience, but it is vital that in an interview setting you are able to communicate this to the panel.

In order to achieve this you need to prepare well. This will enable you to achieve the following:
- Anticipate the questions
- Prepare your answers
- Practise your answers.

Preparing interview answers in advance

It is important to be aware of potential interview questions for two main reasons:
- When you are asked a question that you already anticipated being asked, it does not produce the typical 'shell-shocked' response that usually presents as an unimpressive time delay. Even if you do not have a pre-prepared answer, the response of your brain and body will be more natural and your recovery time will be quicker when answering a question that you had anticipated.
- More importantly, if you are prepared, you will be able to think in advance why the question has been asked and what reply is most appropriate. You may even be able to recite a reply from memory although, in our opinion, it is better not to produce a clearly scripted answer straight from a textbook, since it often appears less considered or thoughtful. It is relatively easy for interviewers to spot a candidate reciting an answer word for word, and there is always the danger that you may forget your script.

How to prepare your answers

If you are answering a question such as **'Why do you want to be a Surgeon?'** the best approach is to consider a few key reasons, and prepare them in your mind as a series of bullet-points. Bearing in mind that interviewers allow approximately 3 minutes per question (including asking the question and probing), you should aim to get across just two or three key messages rather than 20.

You will score higher in the interview if you can demonstrate a good understanding of a topic. The best way to do this is with personal examples. If you are asked to describe **'What is meant by clinical governance?'**, then choose an answer that highlights an example from your own clinical practice.

This will be far more impressive than if you were to regurgitate the standard definition.

By accurately predicting the questions you are going to be asked at interview, you will give more considered and sensible replies. It is worth remembering that most questions are asked for a reason. Most often the interviewer is examining your experience, your knowledge, your skills, your attitude and your personality. As part of your preparation, take time to consider the reasons why each question gets asked at interview.

Some great news: '90% of interview questions are entirely predictable'.

You should aim to construct a list of likely questions based upon the information given in this book. You then need to prepare your answers and practise them.

There are potentially hundreds of possible questions, and interviewers will always be able to think up new ones. It will not be possible to prepare a set answer to every possible question. However, by thinking about the common/predictable questions, and having a good level of understanding of the key topics, you will have more confidence walking in to the interview.

Practising answers

It is important to practise answering questions out loud. The easiest and least embarrassing option is to practise speaking to walls and mirrors. This can be a useful way of planning how you structure answers in your mind, and you can time your answers. Better still, you could video yourself. Be aware, however, that without someone else providing feedback, you are likely to reinforce mistakes and bad habits.

The best way to practise answering questions is by organising a mock interview. If your current most senior colleague is helpful, you could ask whether he or she would be willing to interview you formally. Alternatively, a group of more junior colleagues may be willing to stage a mock interview. This can make the real thing a little less intimidating, and gives you the chance to get constructive feedback. Some departments or GP surgeries may even have video facilities. If yours does, take advantage of this so you can observe your body language, speech patterns and any nervous habits you may possess.

Interview courses

There are a number of interview skills courses available. It is worth considering attending a course if you want to get an edge at interview. They are particularly helpful for more nervous individuals since increased preparation is associated with increased confidence. When you are investigating available courses, try to find out how many other people will be on the course with you. Those courses with fewer attendees may be more useful since they are more likely to provide individualised one-to-one feedback.

Medical interview courses on the web

- www.medical-interviews.co.uk
- www.apply2medicine.co.uk
- www.medicalcommunicationskills.com
- www.interview-intelligence.com

2.8 Your appearance at interview

Depending on your source, you are likely to hear conflicting advice about what to wear at interview. As a general rule you should look smart and professional. This is true for all interviews, regardless of seniority and specialty. Your interviewers are likely to be quite conservative in their attitude and expectations, so if in doubt select conservative attire yourself and resist the temptation to dress extravagantly.

Gentlemen

Decide in advance what suit you are going to wear. Opt for a dark, smart suit. Check if it needs a trip to the dry-cleaners as a result of a food fight at the last wedding you attended. Select either a white, pale blue or beige shirt. Select a fairly plain tie that doesn't draw too much attention. Generally, the wearing of old school ties is not recommended. Your shoes should be of good quality but, most importantly, polished.

Finally, pay attention to your grooming. Do you need a haircut? Are your nails clipped? Have you shaved? It is probably best to avoid potent aftershave.

Ladies

As your objective is to look smart and professional, the safest option is to wear trousers. If you choose to wear a dress or a skirt, the choice of length is a personal decision. Avoid anything too revealing, since you may alienate conservative panel members (both male and female). Opt for a plain blouse or shirt (e.g. pink or beige). Wear shoes that are smart and comfortable. Avoid, if possible, excessive make-up, jewellery and pungent perfume.

2.9　Arriving at the interview

Think about how you are going to get to the interview on time to avoid a last minute panic. If you will have a long distance to travel, then consider staying in a hotel or with friends the night before.

If you are travelling on the day, make sure you allow plenty of time for travelling by train or by road. If you are driving, find out about parking beforehand.

2.10　Final interview preparation

Interviews often run late, and you are likely to arrive early. You may therefore have a long wait. To counteract this, you could spend time talking to the other candidates, but this can add to your stress levels. Speaking to someone who has already been interviewed can be very useful, however, as you might be able to find out what questions are being asked. If you are sure how long the delay is, then one alternative is to take a short walk and get some fresh air.

Make sure that you take a toilet break before your interview. Ensure that you have had something to eat and drink too.

Rehearse the very likely questions but don't get too worked up. Think positive thoughts. Remind yourself of previous interview successes and what a great doctor you are, and hopefully you will walk in the interview room with confidence and a smile on your face.

2.11 Summary

You should prepare well in advance of your interview. Here is a checklist to remind you of the key components of interview preparation:

Interview preparation checklist

- Get to know yourself, your strengths and your weaknesses
- Be able to talk about everything on your CV/application form
- Look at the Deanery website, and the Trust/Hospital/General Practice websites (if relevant)
- Consider making an informal visit
- Consider asking someone to 'put in a good word' for you in advance
- Be aware of training and future developments in your chosen specialty, and get experience
- Be able to talk about a recent journal article you have read or NICE/NSF guidelines relevant to your specialty.
- Think about the questions in advance and a framework for answering them
- Practise interview skills and consider going on a course
- Have a look at www.bbc.co.uk/health for recent health topics in the news
- Plan what you are going to wear and your transport in advance
- Read the remaining chapters of this book!

Chapter 3 **Performing at the interview**

3.1 Introduction

This chapter covers some of the key areas that relate to performance during the medical interview. We cover areas of interview etiquette that include how to make the most of your introduction and departure and how to communicate effectively in between. We also give guidance and suggestions for dealing with the final, anxiety-inducing question: 'Is there anything you would like to ask us?'

3.2 First impressions

Traditionally, the interview process has been structured as a one-off meeting with an interview panel. With the advent of assessment centres, the interview structure has altered. Some interviews comprise a number of different stations, each with a smaller number of interviewers or assessors. For candidates that are well prepared, this can be advantageous since it enables you to make a good first impression on several occasions. It is essential to ascertain the structure of your interview in advance so that you can prepare effectively.

Initially a member of the interview panel or a representative from Medical Personnel will call you in to the interview room.

You should seize the opportunity to make a good first impression. As you walk through the door, smile and acknowledge all of the panel members. If panel members approach you, then give a small nod, greet them with a 'hello' and shake hands with everyone. Do not ignore any Medical Personnel representatives or observers that might be present.

Remember a good firm handshake but not so firm as to cause any physical discomfort!

How to Succeed at the Medical Interview By C. Smith and D. Meeking. 2008 by Blackwell Publishing, ISBN: 978-1-4051-6729-1.

Wait until you are asked to sit down or, if this instruction does not appear to be forthcoming, ask if it is all right to take a seat.

Where a large interview panel is present, there will usually be an initial greeting and an introduction to the other panel members by the chairperson. In this scenario, each panel member may be introduced to you more formally. It may be appropriate to shake the hands of each panel member across the desk, but more frequently there will be a nod of recognition from each. The key here is to reciprocate as appropriate. Do not force the panel members to shake your hand when it is clear that this is not expected!

If the interview process involves rotating through different stations, it may not be appropriate to shake hands with your assessors at each stage. Again, it is best to reciprocate as guided by your interviewer/assessor.

One example of where hand shaking is inappropriate would be where you are taking part in a group discussion with other candidates as part of a GP selection process. The large number of candidates and assessors makes the process too time-consuming for formal greetings. In any case, the objective of these exercises is to observe your interaction with your peers, rather than your assessors.

As a general rule, greet and shake hands with your interviewers if you will be interacting with them, otherwise just do as you are asked!

In the traditional interview setting, you will be seated and then may receive a polite enquiry as to how far you have travelled. The early enquiries are often deliberately chosen to help you settle and put you at your ease. Do not reply with a long wordy account of your travels. After this brief exchange, the interview proper will commence and you will be asked a series of questions.

If you have come straight from night duty, it is worth briefly mentioning this fact since it can have a moderating effect on aggressive questioning from some panel members.

3.3 Effective communication

It has been suggested that about 60% of our communication relates to body language, 30% to the method of delivery and only 10% to the language.

What does this mean? Well, it means that you should pay attention to your body language and the way that you deliver information rather than simply the factual content of your answers.

Body language

You should seat yourself in an open posture. This means sitting with your hands rested on your lap. Avoid the temptation to sit with your arms folded since this gives the impression of being defensive. This should not be surprising or new information for you, but it remains surprisingly common to see interviewed doctors adopting closed, defensive positions.

You should sit upright. Do not slouch! If you feel more comfortable, you can cross your legs. Try to sit quietly still and wait for the first question.

As you are being asked the first question you can lean in slightly. Look the questioner in the eye. This way you are being seen to be listening and taking an interest. Remember to look away periodically to avoid appearing threatening.

An interviewer's perspective

The warm, confident, smart and attractive individual who oozes professionalism and engages the interviewer in a comfortable, slick manner without betraying a hint of nervousness is more likely to succeed. The quiet, fidgety and unconfident individual who stares at their chewed fingernails whilst mumbling unintelligibly to the panel is less likely to return home happy.

Delivering your answers

Take a moment before you start to answer the question. Primarily direct your answer towards the questioner, but try to include all of the members of the interview panel in your answer. This means obtaining eye contact with the questioner but occasionally moving your head and sweeping your eyes gently around to the rest of the panel. Try to keep everybody's attention. Your objective should be to gain the support of all panel members.

Try to use gentle hand movements and vary the tone of your voice. Monotonous voices will tend to lose the panel's attention rather quickly, since they may have been interviewing for several hours before you appeared in the room.

3.4 Selling yourself

Reveal your personality

It is important that you try to enjoy the interview experience. This will allow your personality to show. Do not attempt to make jokes if this is not something that you are usually comfortable doing. If you do decide to give a humorous answer, it is best that it is self-deprecating, i.e. that you are the butt of the humour rather than others. Gentle spontaneous humour can have a positive effect on interview outcome, since it suggests an enjoyable engaging process. It also allows panel members a glimpse into your non-interview persona.

Needless to say you should avoid loud, bawdy or raucous comments that might alienate your interviewers. Only use language and context that you would use in polite company.

In general, if you are asked your personal opinion on a subject matter, for example your views on the role of Nurse Consultants, then you should express your own beliefs. This will appear natural and believable. However, always remember that your beliefs should be tempered by the beliefs of others, particularly panel members! If you do have strong, controversial ideas on some subjects, it can be better to tone these down in an interview situation to avoid conflict. This is particularly true if you don't have a full grasp of the issues.

You need to demonstrate that you are capable of independent thought, but are not so truculent that you will cause trouble with your colleagues who have different viewpoints from your own.

Be diplomatic, and try to demonstrate a good understanding of all the issues. Importantly, and wherever possible, you should indicate that a conflicting idea has some merit.

Be professional

A professional demeanour can be displayed through an appropriate appearance (see Chapter 2). More evidence of your professionalism occurs when you demonstrate that you can interact appropriately with other people (see 'first impressions' earlier).

The way to confirm your professionalism is through being able to talk confidently about your career and issues that relate to your specialty, and by answering questions that test your knowledge and generic skills (see Chapters 5 and 6).

Be confident

Confidence should come with effective preparation. If you have had previous interview successes, try to focus on those achievements. If you have not, then focus upon your career achievements and the efforts you have made in preparing for the interview. Importantly, focus on yourself and do not waste energy thinking about your competition.

You should be clear in your mind why you are the best person for the job. After that, get in there, be yourself and try to enjoy it!

Above all else, be yourself!

3.5 Answering questions

There are several important themes to consider when answering interview questions. These are listed below.

Be concise

It is important to answer questions concisely. Nervousness most commonly leads to long waffling responses. You should aim to be calm and measured in your replies. Don't be tempted to fill every break in conversation with more words.

Slow down

You should also avoid speaking too quickly. This is a common problem at interview and can be avoided by a few practice sessions in front of a mirror.

Always take a moment to compose yourself before starting your answer. Think about the question and the key points that you want to get across. As previously stated, aim to keep the length of your answer below 2 minutes.

Talk about yourself

If you get asked a question such as 'Tell me about your last audit', you should talk specifically about your own role, rather than 'we did this and we did that . . .'. You are then conveying to the panel a personal and active role in the audit. It gives you a chance to highlight your organisational and administrative skills, and shows that you can perform as part of a team.

Give personal examples

Whenever possible, demonstrate your understanding of a subject by giving a personal example. For example, if you were asked 'What is meant by professional integrity?', you could highlight an example of when you had to take responsibility for a particular action you had taken. (There is a section on answering questions asking for examples in Chapter 6.)

Be objective

Try to back up your statements with evidence. For example, in response to the difficult question 'Are you a good communicator?' you could mention that you have active listening skills, and include evidence from your latest 360-degree appraisal, that highlighted this as a positive attribute.

3.6 Coping with the question that you don't understand

You may be asked a question that you do not understand. This can happen for a number of reasons:

- Perhaps you did not hear all of the interviewer's words or the interviewer spoke too quietly. Maybe you are a little hard of hearing or were too nervous to concentrate properly.

Dealing with this scenario is simple. Just reply: 'I'm terribly sorry, I didn't quite catch that, could you repeat the question please?'

- The interviewer may use a word that you are not familiar with. This can happen more frequently if English is not your first language.

For this scenario the reply should be 'I'm sorry, could you please rephrase the question?' This should avoid the same wording.

- You could be asked a question that you feel completely unable to answer because you have no knowledge of the subject matter. For example 'What did you think about the BMA's recent response to the latest GMC proposal on dealing with negligent doctors?' or 'What are your opinions on the role of the Healthcare Commission?'

If your immediate thought is 'I haven't got a clue' then don't panic! If you honestly have no idea how to answer the question, then nothing will be gained by trying to make something up.

Try this as a reply, 'Sorry, I am not aware of those comments, could you tell me what they were?' or 'Sorry, I don't know what the role of the Healthcare Commission is, could you please tell me?' This way you are showing interest as well as still having a chance to contribute to the discussion after being helped in the right direction.

It might even be possible to demonstrate that you do have some knowledge of related areas even where you cannot directly answer the question. For example, 'I am not aware of those comments, although this is a rather turbulent time for the GMC since the Harold Shipman investigation. There is a lot of governmental pressure to reform and I suspect there may be frequent clashes between the GMC and the BMA in response to proposed changes'.

If you feel unable to deflect the questions or do not feel that any of the above suggestions are appropriate, then give a simple honest response, such as, 'I am afraid I am not familiar with this'. This answer will enable the interviewer to expand upon the question or, better still, to ask a different question.

3.7 'Do you have any questions for us?'

This is the question that is most commonly asked at the end of your interview. There are two ways to approach your answer.

Option 1 — When you do not have any questions to ask

It is important when choosing this response to demonstrate that there are good reasons why you do not need to ask any questions. An example answer might be:

> 'No thank you, I have had the opportunity of meeting several members of the interview panel prior to the interview and all of my questions have been answered.'

or

'No thank you, I have had the opportunity to meet with a number of colleagues who are currently in post and they have answered all of the questions that I had.'

For additional emphasis, your answer could be supported with evidence. For example:

'I have had the chance to ask about the in-house educational programme, and I was encouraged when I was told that previous trainees have had good success with the FRCS exam.'

The argument for using option 1 as a reply is that you shouldn't ask a question that you really should have found the answer to before the interview. It might indicate that you haven't done your research. In reality, however, interviewers do not expect that it is possible for all of your questions to be answered in advance.

If you choose not to ask any questions, then make it clear to the interview panel that you have researched the post.

Option 2 — When you have genuine questions to ask

It is not unreasonable to ask questions at the end of the interview. In fact most interviewers expect it. It is vital, however, that you ask appropriate questions. There are numerous examples of candidates spoiling their chances at the last minute by asking dumb or inappropriate questions.

Do not ask questions that you clearly should have found out the answers to prior to the interview, for example 'What specialty will I be working in?' or 'How long does the post last for?', unless these details have bizarrely been missed out in the advertisement or job description.

Do not ask inappropriate questions. Specifically, the subjects of annual leave and pay should be avoided. These questions should be asked separately to the interview. Don't run the risk of appearing to be greedy or work-shy immediately prior to leaving the interview room.

Here are a number of questions that are neither dumb nor inappropriate:

- I have enjoyed teaching medical students in my previous posts. What opportunities are there for teaching in this post?
- I have a special interest in x or y. Do any of the Consultants/Partners have any special interests?
- I am planning to work towards my MRCP in the next 2 years. Have previous trainees here enjoyed exam success?

- I completed an audit in my last post. Are there any on-going audits or research opportunities that I could get involved with here?

Of course, you could find out the answers to all of these questions before the interview. But by asking questions in this way, it firstly demonstrates your experience and interests, and, secondly, conveys enthusiasm, giving the impression that you intend to contribute to the post.

3.8 How to end the interview

Last impressions can be as important as first impressions!

Irrespective of how well or badly you think the interview has gone, follow the same departure routine. Stand up, shake hands if offered, and smile. Thank each member of the interview panel individually if it is a small group. Thank the whole panel if it is a large group, and leave.

It should have been made clear beforehand whether you are expected to wait around to hear if you are successful. Often you will be allowed to leave, and will subsequently be contacted by phone or e-mail, as indicated by the panel or in advance of the interview.

If you are offered the opportunity to stay behind and are able to do so, you should stay. This should give you the opportunity of receiving vital personal feedback if you have been unsuccessful.

3.9 Feedback

You may not have been successful at this interview. Sometimes there are just too many good candidates. Whatever you think the reason might be, take the opportunity to get feedback from the people that interviewed you. This is invaluable and if they are being honest you will get important information to help you prepare for your next interview. You will need to identify areas of weakness at interview or gaps in your CV that need to be improved. It also indicates to the interviewers that you are disappointed and shows that you are keen to improve. This may help you if you apply for the same post in the future.

If you fail at interview then as well as asking why you were unsuccessful, you should ask about the strengths of the successful candidate.

3.10 Summary

Do:
- Greet the panel members individually
- Sit with an open posture

- Try to convey confidence, professionalism and your true personality
- Think carefully about what questions (if any) to ask at the end
- Be yourself
- Obtain feedback if you are unsuccessful.

Don't:

- Slouch and fold your arms
- Ignore the Medical Personnel representative
- Be afraid to admit if you don't understand the question
- Express very controversial opinions
- Ask questions about pay and annual leave.

Chapter 4 **Common interview questions**

4.1 Introduction

The aim of this chapter is to tell you those interview questions that will frequently be asked and to give you tips as to how you should answer them. It is important to expect these questions and to prepare thoroughly for them.

There are always inevitable questions in any interview process. The key to success is to prepare for them well. By making the most of these predictable questions you will significantly improve your chances of success.

Interviewers will want to know about you, your experience, and your motivation in applying for the post.

4.2 Questions about you

In the early stages of a traditional medical interview it is very common to be asked questions that relate directly to you, your background, your experience and your personality. Questions can be fairly open such as 'Tell us about yourself', or they be more specific such as 'How well do you communicate with others?'

Being prepared for these questions in advance will help you score highly at the interview. We have included a number of likely questions with tips that will enable you to provide effective answers.

'Tell us about yourself and your career so far'

This is a common open-ended question that gives you a wonderful opportunity to sell yourself. It is a good question to be asked because it enables you, with a carefully constructed answer, to score points in a number of different areas. The most common mistakes when answering this question are stumbling because you don't know where to start or waffling through your entire CV.

How to Succeed at the Medical Interview By C. Smith and D. Meeking. 2008 by Blackwell Publishing, ISBN: 978-1-4051-6729-1.

Also be wary about focusing too much on one area of specific interest, i.e. this is not a licence to spend 15 minutes talking about your success in clay pigeon shooting competitions!

Here is an example answer:

'I am 30 years old and from Somerset originally. I trained at Cardiff Medical School. After my house officer posts I completed 6 months of A&E in Bournemouth before working as an expedition doctor in Belize for 3 months. On returning to the UK I entered a 3-year medical rotation and successfully completed my MRCP. Over the past 9 months I have worked at Registrar level in Cardiology. During this time I was actively involved in audit projects, MRCP and Medical student teaching, and made several presentations at regional meetings.

I then went to work as a doctor with Médicins Sans Frontières in Uganda for 6 months. Here I gained exposure to Paediatrics and Tropical diseases, as well as management and administrative experience.

I have many interests outside of work, including sailing and a range of sporting activities, as well as spending time with my friends and family.

I have decided on a career in General Practice because I enjoy a variety of work and dealing with patients of all ages and being able to offer continuation of care.

In my professional and social life I have developed skills that enable me to communicate well with others and work effectively as part of a team.

In the future I would like to be a General Practitioner with a special interest in Cardiovascular medicine.'

This answer highlights a number of different areas that interviewers will be interested to hear about. These areas include clinical experience, exam success, enthusiasm for teaching and audit, generic skills and motivation for General Practice. It also indicates that you have an interesting life away from medicine.

You should be able to produce a similar answer that you can present in less than 2 minutes.

It is essential to make the most of open questions such as this. It is likely that subsequent questions will focus more specifically on certain aspects that you raised in your response to this question.

Rather than trying to rehearse answers word for word, it is better to use a 'mental framework' for your replies. This enables you to provide thoughtful and flexible answers to specific questions. The following is a framework that you might use:

- Summarise your clinical and academic experience — just the highlights
- Mention your other generic skills (for more on this see Chapter 6)
- Highlight activities outside of medicine
- Include your personal motivation for the post and give an indication of where you see yourself in the future.

Don't go into too much detail about any one area. Just try to cover each of these areas.

Practise your answers out loud to close friends or the bathroom mirror.

'What personal qualities do you possess?' or 'Why should we appoint you?'

This question appears at first to be quite different, but careful inspection reveals that the interviewer is looking for similar information to the previous question. This time, however, the focus is less on your professional career to date and more on your personality.

You can still use the same framework to answer this question, but adapt it to highlight your more personal qualities.

'In all of my previous posts I have been told that I am conscientious, knowledgeable and that my work is appreciated. I have evidence of this from my appraisal reports and thank-you letters that I have received from patients. I am enthusiastic and have involved myself in audit projects and MRCP teaching, and I have also given several clinical presentations at regional specialty meetings.

Having worked in a number of different hospital settings in the UK and in Uganda with Médicins Sans Frontières, I have shown that I can adapt to different working environments. Many of my posts have involved working closely within a team setting. This has increased my communication and teamworking skills. Working with MSF gave me some management experience since I had the responsibility of looking after more than one hundred staff. I also gained useful financial experience in managing a drug budget.

In general I know that I am hard working and work well with patients and colleagues. I balance my work life by enjoying myself away from the workplace. I enjoy spending time with my friends and family, as well as being a keen sailor and participating in other sports.

I want to be a GP because I enjoy seeing patients from different backgrounds with a wide variety of clinical conditions. I also feel interested and confident in the administrative and management aspects of the role.'

When giving answers to these open-ended questions, it is important not to simply make statements about your own skills, but back them up by using examples of your experience and evidence from previous feedback you have obtained. This serves two purposes: firstly it makes your answers more convincing, and secondly you are able to score more points by highlighting your achievements.

An answer like this is much more powerful than a standard one such as 'I am a good team-player and I have great communication skills'.

Where is the evidence to back up your statement? Try to stand out from the crowd by giving evidence provided by feedback and experience!

'Where do you see yourself in 5 years' time?'

As you study each of these questions you will notice that they are not as different from each other as they first appear. Again you can use our example framework for answering this question, only this time the focus is more on your future plans.

Once again you must highlight examples from a variety of settings to support your chosen career; the details will depend upon your experience and the specialty to which you are applying.

When you talk about where you see yourself in the future you should be honest and attempt to present a clear vision. Even if you are uncertain, try and present a limited number of possibilities. You should not, under any circumstances, simply say that you are unsure or that you don't know. This suggests that you don't care or haven't considered the question.

Bear in mind that the interview panel might have certain expectations for the future of successful candidates.

Therefore, with interviews for senior medical posts you should be expecting (and wanting, for the purposes of the interview) to have an interest in roles that are relevant to that post. This might include management, teaching or service development roles.

'Give us three adjectives that describe you best'

This appears to be a trickier version of an earlier question. Don't get too hung up on the adjectives, but think through why the question is being asked. When contemplating your reply, think to yourself, 'What are the qualities of a good doctor?' or, better still, 'What are my qualities?' The answers should lie within the framework you have considered for answering questions of this type. Be able to justify your answers by giving evidence with examples from your experience or feedback. For example:

> 'Three adjectives that I would use to describe myself are assertive, enthusiastic and organised. When I was a medical SHO studying for the MRCP I set up a study group and arranged regular daily teaching which resulted in most of our group passing the exam . . .'

'How do you rate your communication skills?'

Think about what the hallmarks of good communication skills are (see Chapter 6). 'Strong' is a good adjective to use to describe your active listening and communicating skills. Back up your statement by giving evidence from 360-degree appraisals, supportive comments from colleagues and thank-you letters that you have received.

'What are your main strengths?'

When preparing a framework to answer this question, think of five strengths, backed up with evidence and examples. Try not to focus on just one strength. You can use the same examples as you did for the previous question.

If you are struggling to think of strengths then take a look at the Person Specifications for the post, see which requirements are most relevant to you, and think of examples that demonstrate your abilities in these areas.

For more senior medical posts it is important that you highlight your clinical knowledge and expertise as strengths. Good communication skills are also essential, and it is worth thinking of one or two examples that highlight your strength in this area.

'What is your main weakness?'

This is a question that everybody dreads and can be a difficult question to answer. It is worth contemplating why an interview panel would want to pose this question.

Primarily, this question is asked to gain a deeper understanding of an individual's personality and to gauge whether the candidate is capable of honest, open and personal discussion. After all, this is a skill that might be important when dealing with emotional issues concerning patients and their families.

The question also confirms to an examiner that a candidate has some insight into personal failings. Without insight, there can presumably be no personal improvement.

It is important, however, that the weaknesses you state do not frighten your interview panel, and there are therefore a limited number of weaknesses that you should admit to in an interview situation!

Another way to approach this question is to think of it as a *strength gone too far*. Try to think of an example of a personal characteristic that you like but that has somehow got you into trouble. Perversely, by turning the weakness back into a strength, you can escape relatively unscathed, and even endear yourelf to the interview panel if the answer is delivered with a wry smile.

Let's imagine for instance that you like to phone colleagues at the Hospital after work to check on sick patients that you have handed over towards the end of a shift. On one occasion your patient's condition may have worsened and you spent the next 20 minutes filling in your colleague with more details about the patient and as a result missed the start of the film you were going to watch at the cinema. Your weakness is that you sometimes find it difficult to switch off, even though you understand that this is unhealthy. It would be sensible to follow this example by saying that you have changed your practice so that you no longer ring your colleagues after work unless you think it is important.

The most common response to this difficult question is to talk about how you pay too much attention to detail and find it difficult to delegate tasks to others. This is another way of suggesting that you are a perfectionist. (Please avoid saying 'I am too much of a perfectionist'.) It may be best to steer clear of this answer altogether. It has been used so many times that it has lost its sincerity and its believability.

If you are worried about giving an honest answer you can always temper your response by indicating that you are rectifying your fault. For instance:

'When I first started working in out-patient clinics, I struggled to take a focused history and got lost in the detail of chronic ailments. I have since spent time sitting in with more senior colleagues to discover how they deal with this problem and now I feel much more confident and I make much more effective use of clinic time.'

The same principle applies when talking about mistakes you have made. You should indicate that you have corrected, or are in the process of correcting, personal failings.

'Why should we recruit you rather than another candidate?'

This question is similar to the earlier question 'What are your main strengths?' and should be answered in a similar fashion. Make sure that you avoid criticising your competition. Simply concentrate on selling yourself. You can begin your answer with:

'I am sure there are many good candidates being interviewed today. This is what I have to offer you . . .'

'What is your greatest/proudest/most memorable achievement?'

It is worth thinking about this beforehand. If phrased in this way it should not matter whether you choose a medical or a non-medical achievement. Give a brief account of the achievement and explain why it was important to you. You may also use this as an opportunity to demonstrate what you have gained and how you have learnt from the experience.

For instance, if you choose to mention that it was winning the county Badminton Championship, you might add that this has improved your confidence. Or, if it was the birth of your first child, you could mention that this has improved the value you attach to life or heightened your awareness of the patient experience.

'Tell us about your hobbies/interests (and how do they influence your medical practice?)'

Hobby-related questions are common. They are chosen because they give the candidate an opportunity to relax and interact in a less formal manner. Think carefully when listing hobbies and interests on your CV, and be prepared to demonstrate your knowledge and enthusiasm about them.

It is important to bear in mind that many senior doctors are fairly conservative, so it is probably best to leave out hobbies and interests that are too unconventional or unhealthy. Mentioning on-line gambling or pub crawls is a no-no! Sports and musical interests are usually are a safer bet!

Sometimes you can be asked how a particular hobby relates to your work. This is a good opportunity to highlight some generic skills. For example:

'As the captain of the Junior Doctors Cricket team I arrange a number of fixtures and am involved in team selection. I have found this organisational and leadership experience to be extremely useful in the workplace.'

Think of a hobby or interest where you utilise one of the following skills, and consider how it positively influences you at work:
- Team-playing
- Leadership
- Organisational
- Management
- Communication
- Coping with pressure.

There is a range of similar questions that you may be asked. Remember that if you have a framework for answering these questions they should be easy point-scorers for you.

Some commonly asked questions that relate to YOU

- 'What personal attributes do you have that would make you a good Ophthalmologist/General Practitioner/Obstetrician?'
- 'How would your friends describe you?'
- 'Have you ever received feedback directly from your patients?'
- 'What did you learn during your last post?'
- 'What do you have to offer us?'

4.3 Questions that test your motivation and commitment to the specialty

'Why do you want to work in this Trust/Hospital/city/region?'

All of us will have different reasons for applying for posts. In addition to professional or career motivation, there are often personal, social or financial considerations. When answering this question it is sensible to mention each of these, with the exception of financial motivation. You should talk about professional and career motives before your personal and social reasons. Again it is important to have considered this question prior to interview so that you can research and properly structure your response.

Professional and career motives

If you are an external candidate then, where appropriate, you should demonstrate that you have researched the local Deanery and relevant departments. If you are an internal candidate, then your familiarity will give you an advantage. If not, then by familiarising yourself with your new environment you will be able to use this information when answering questions.

For instance:

> 'I visited the department 2 weeks ago and met with several of the Consultants. I was very impressed with the quality of the training programme offered here.'

Regardless of whether you are an internal candidate or not, you should familiarise yourself with any relevant Hospital, Trust or Practice websites. Try to read a report from the Healthcare Commission if you can. Find something that could impress and flatter the interview panel, for example:

> 'This Trust has a reputation for high quality of care. I see from your website that the Trust has a very proactive strategy towards combating MRSA infection, and that you have achieved a reduction in cases in the past 2 years.'

Flattery, provided it is not overdone, will serve you well. Positive comments about the department's reputation will warm the panel towards you, but try to be specific to achieve maximum credibility. Again you can use this question to demonstrate that you have researched the post thoroughly:

> 'The current post holders are very enthusiastic about the quality of the training programme, and trainees have enjoyed a high success rate in postgraduate examinations.'

It is worth following up positive comments about a department, Trust or Deanery by demonstrating how this matches your own strengths and aspirations. Furthermore, you may wish to describe how you might contribute to the department.

For senior posts, you will impress the panel by focusing upon the Trust as a whole. You can highlight areas of excellence within the Trust that match your own interests, and can focus upon Trust strategy and the contribution you can make to this.

Personal and social motives

You may have chosen to apply for a post because your partner works in the area and is unable to relocate. Perhaps you like living in big cities. Maybe the Hospital you are choosing is by the sea and you are a keen sailor. These are all valid reasons, and you should not be too concerned about highlighting them. Just don't mention them first!

A carefully thought out answer may be very beneficial to you. It could lead the interviewer towards a series of benign questions about things that interest you. This will help you to relax and enable you to discuss topics that might endear you to your interview panel.

'Why are you applying for this specialty?'

This question is very likely to be asked at interviews for ST posts or General Practice. It is essential that you research this question prior to interview (see Chapter 2). When answering, you need to demonstrate clearly that you have fully investigated and have acquired a depth of knowledge about your chosen specialty. An effective technique in answering this question is first to consider the pros and cons of the specialty, thus enabling you to give a carefully thought out and balanced answer.

Common explanations for career choices

Reasons to pursue a career in Surgery:
- It is a practical, 'hands-on' specialty and I enjoy technical procedures
- I have an interest and knowledge of anatomy

Reasons to pursue a career in General Practice:
- The variety of work is huge
- I can follow up patients and families for life. I enjoy continuity of care
- I have the opportunity to manage people of all ages

Reasons to pursue a career in Hospital Medicine:
- I enjoy helping to make acutely unwell patients better
- I have an analytical mind and enjoy investigating and managing difficult cases
- I enjoy the contact and communication with patients, their friends and family

---

Try to think of 4–6 reasons why you have chosen the particular specialty. Convey enthusiasm as well as a sense of realism and insight, showing that you really do see yourself in the specialty in the future.

Don't, whatever you do, make it sound as if you are only choosing a specialty because the alternatives are worse! Your responses should be positive.

If a post contains the potential for teaching and research, incorporate any interests or experience of this into your response.

To help you answer this predictable question consider the following:
- Why do you find the specialty interesting?
- What can you offer this specialty?
- Where is this specialty likely to be in 5–10 years' time?
- Where do you see yourself in 5–10 years' time?

'Why have you changed direction at this stage in your career?'
Doctors have always switched from one career to another. Even with the more directive training programme associated with the MMC process, people will continue to move away from one career path and towards another. If you do switch careers, you will inevitably be asked for your reasons.

You may be asked because interviewers are suspicious as to your motives, although it is more likely they are genuinely interested in the factors that led to the change. It is important not to adopt a defensive response to this line of questioning.

It is important to avoid giving negative reasons for changing your career path. You should steer clear of certain commonly used statements.

Things not to say:
- 'I am fed up with night shifts'
- 'I didn't enjoy my previous job'
- 'I had to get out of Hospital Medicine'

   Instead, focus on the positive reasons for your career change, such as:
- 'I completed a wide variety of medical posts and I enjoyed all the specialties. I particularly enjoyed the variety of people and conditions that I came across in A&E. I have chosen to be a GP because I have an interest and enthusiasm for all areas of Medicine and feel that my previous experience will be valuable'
- 'Although I have trained as a Paediatrician and I enjoy my job immensely, I am not seeing the range of problems I expected to see as a doctor. I would like to be a GP with a special interest in Paediatrics. This way I hope to be able to have a greater variety of work and also continue to care for my patients throughout their lives'

'Why would you like this post?'

If you get asked the more general 'Why this post?' question then you should consider all of the aspects discussed:
- Why this Trust/Hospital/department/city? (see earlier)
- Why this specialty? (see earlier)

   Try to give an answer that incorporates both of these important factors, giving an abbreviated version of each.

   It goes without saying that you should never go for a job interview unless you are sure that you want the post.

   It is surprising how often this rule is ignored. If you are reading this book and preparing for these questions as we suggest, then this shouldn't be the case with you. It usually comes across clearly if applicants don't have a genuine interest in a post. You should always be prepared to accept a post if it is offered to you at interview. If you do not, this may be viewed as wasting the interview panel's time and this might jeopardise attempts to land future posts within the same region or similar specialty.

'What made you choose Medicine as a career?'

Some interviewers like to take you back in time and explore the reasons you chose a medical career in the first place. This is usually because they want to find out a little bit more about your motives and the way you think.

   Avoid the corny response 'because I want to help people' that may have just about succeeded at Medical School interviews. As with all of these questions, aim to convey a few key points, and improvise your answer around this. Remember to base your answer on the truth. Interviewers are likely to see through less genuine responses. You might want to consider the following areas:

- An interest in sciences at school
- Opportunity to combine science with a compassionate profession
- Inspiration from work experience or previous contact with the medical profession.

Other common questions that test your motivation

- 'What do you like and dislike about this specialty?'
- 'What opportunities do you feel that a career in Paediatrics can offer you, and what do you think you can offer it?'
- 'Do you really want this job?'
- 'Would you accept the job if we offered it to you today?'

4.4 Questions that relate to your CV and job experience

Spontaneous unplanned questions may arise during an interview. This might be because panel members have forgotten or are bored with their planned question, or you have already answered it. During the interview, it is probable that interview panel members will be flicking through your CV or application form. Spontaneous unplanned questions will nearly always arise from this scanning.

You will be better prepared to answer questions if you have taken your time to perfect your CV/application form, you know it inside out, and are ready to answer any questions that relate directly to what you have written.

'Talk us through your CV'

This is a common 'ice-breaker' question, designed to give the panel an early feel of your experience and your personality. You obviously should not proceed slowly to talk through your entire CV. If you approach the question in this way you will probably get interrupted at an early stage and will have missed out on a golden opportunity to sell yourself.

You should answer this question in a similar way to 'Tell me about yourself'. Structure your answer so that it follows the order in your CV, since panel members will almost certainly decide to flick through as you are talking. Cover a range of areas, and draw their attention to the selected highlights that most interest them:

- Your education, qualification and awards
- Clinical experience, audits, research, teaching

- Management and administrative experience
- Hobbies and interests
- Your motivation for the job and where you see yourself in the future.

Remember to emphasise the positive aspects of your CV that set you apart from others.

'Why did you take 2 years out of Medicine?'

There is some concern as to whether this should be a legitimate question at interview. Enthusiastic Medical Personnel representatives or experienced panel members may ban this question. It might be construed as disadvantaging applicants who took a career break for health or personal reasons, but there can be no doubt that it is still asked, and for that reason we have included it in this book. Interviewers may be suspicious of career gaps. You should be prepared to justify them with honest answers. Frequent explanations are travel, difficulty obtaining work, building up finances with locum work, health and personal reasons.

Tell the truth and then move on!

For example:

'I had a desire to explore Central America while I was still young. I carried out some locum work for 6 months to build up enough money to travel then spent 12 months in the deserts of Southern Mexico. It was a fantastic experience that I will always look back on fondly.

It gave me time to consider my career options and on my return I applied for a specialist training post in Dermatology since I had always had an interest in skin disease . . . etc.'

'What is the most exceptional part of your CV?'

This question is a variation on the theme of 'What is your greatest achievement?', 'What is your proudest moment?', etc. Aim to prepare one medical and one non-medical example of your lifetime achievements before you enter the interview room. Medical examples might include completing a PhD or a particular research project, passing a tough exam or perhaps developing a great relationship with a medical team or a patient's family. Non-medical examples could include sporting achievements or important personal milestones (the birth of a child or a marriage).

'Tell me about the presentation you gave at the diabetes conference'

If you get asked about a presentation you have made, consider the following points:

- What was the name of the meeting?
- What type of meeting was it? For example, regional, national or international.
- What were the key points of your presentation?
- How was your presentation received? What feedback did you get?

'What audit projects have you undertaken?'

Create a folder containing any audit projects you have completed. For each audit, prepare a short summary, with bullet points:
- The name of the audit.
- Why did you choose to do the audit?
- Were you working alone or in a team (talk about your contribution, but this is also a chance to highlight teamwork).
- What standards did you use?
- What was your methodology and how did you present your findings?
- What, if any, changes were implemented?
- What measures were taken to complete the audit cycle?

By answering the question in this way, you are also demonstrating your knowledge of audit (for more about audit and research see Chapter 5).

'Tell me about your research'

If you have any research experience, you are very likely to be asked about it at interview. As with audit, make sure that you can easily summarise your research, and make it understandable to the audience.

Consider the following subheadings:
- What was the purpose of the research?
- Who else was involved? (Highlight teamwork)
- How much of it was your work?
- How long did you spend on it? How did you organise your time?
- How was it funded?
- What were your findings and how did you present them?
- Can you quote the titles of any papers that resulted from your work?

'Why do you not have any research experience?'

This might be a problem when applying for more senior positions. You should try to turn this apparent deficit on your CV into a strength. Your options include the following:
- If you think hard enough, you may be able to recall that you have contributed to research projects over the years without actually being listed as an author.
- You can talk about how the main focus of your career to date has been on clinical medicine but you are enthusiastic about doing research in the future (assuming this is true).

• Alternatively, you could say that the main focus of your career to date has been on clinical medicine and, if you are NOT enthusiastic about doing research in the future, supplement this with something else. For instance, you may have a commitment to educating doctors or students. You may alternatively have an interest in developing some aspect of a department's service or you may be enthusiastic about auditing a departmental activity. Tailor your answer to something that the panel will find attractive or necessary.

'What Information Technology (IT) experience do you have?'

This question is asked increasingly often at interviews. Think about IT in three areas, and structure your answer accordingly:
• Basic: Word, PowerPoint, Excel
• Web based: internet, e-mail, website design
• Hospital based: PACS (which stands for Picture Archive Computer System), APEX, etc.

Other common questions about your past experience

• 'Tell us about your career to date'
• 'What teaching have you carried out?'
• 'What teaching methods do you use?'
• 'What courses have you been on?'
• 'Why do you like teaching?'

4.5 Questions about your portfolio

You are likely to be asked to show your portfolio or record of training. Don't forget to take it and have it immediately to hand.

One of the interviewers is likely to spend time looking through and asking questions about your portfolio.

It is vital that you are familiar with everything that is contained within your portfolio.

You may be asked for your opinion on aspects of your portfolio. In addition to questions about audit and research (detailed earlier), the following are commonly asked:
• 'How did you find the mini-CEX experience?'
• 'Do you think mini-DOPS is a useful assessment tool?'
• 'What is your experience and opinion of 360-degree appraisal?'

4.6 Summary

- Preparation in a few key areas will enable you to answer a wide range of questions.
- Create a mental 'filing cabinet' of several answers that might cover the range of questions about your strengths and weaknesses, personal attributes, motivation and skills. You can then select an appropriate reply depending upon the question asked.
- Take full advantage of open-ended 'ice-breaker' questions to sell yourself and cover a range of strengths.
- Give examples wherever possible to back up your statements.
- Be positive and enthusiastic about what you can contribute to the job.
- Know yourself, the post you are applying for, your CV and your portfolio inside out!

Chapter 5 **Interview questions that test your knowledge**

5.1 Introduction

The aim of this chapter is to give examples of questions that test your knowledge and to provide you with the information that you will need to answer these.

Definitions are incorporated to aid your understanding of topics. Try, however, to avoid answers that rely upon textbook definitions described word for word. It is boring for interviewers and it will impress them less than you think.

Instead, you should endeavour to develop an understanding of the topics that you are likely to be asked about and think about how the questions are relevant to you. You can then construct an impressive answer of your own.

A precautionary comment: although some of the topics outlined are fairly timeless, such as questions focusing upon audit and research, other 'hot topics' are always evolving. An obvious current example is MMC. It is highly advisable to look at the references for medical websites provided here, as well as keeping up to date with the mainstream health literature. The *British Medical Journal* (for everyone), the *Lancet* (for Medical specialties), *Hospital Doctor* (for Hospital-based specialties), *Pulse* (for General Practice) and one or two specialty publications will provide a broad spectrum of current medical and political knowledge.

The topics and questions outlined below will be relevant to doctors of all specialties, although your priorities will vary according to your own grade and specialty. You should be well informed about the latest developments relevant to the specialty that you are applying for.

How to Succeed at the Medical Interview By C. Smith and D. Meeking. 2008 by Blackwell Publishing, ISBN: 978-1-4051-6729-1.

5.2 Evidence-based medicine

'What is evidence-based medicine (EBM)?'

The most well-known and widely quoted definition for EBM is:

> The conscientious, explicit, and judicious use of current best
> evidence in making decisions about the care of individual patients.
> The practice of EBM means integrating individual clinical expertise
> with the best available external clinical evidence from systematic
> research.
>
> Sackett DL, Rosenberg WM, Gray JAM. *et al.*

This was revised to a simpler definition in 2000:

> The integration of best research evidence with clinical expertise and
> patient values.
>
> Sackett DL, Rosenberg W, Haynes BR.

Attempting to recite either of these definitions will not, however, serve you well at interview. The first definition is difficult to memorise, and reciting either definition will indicate that you can read a book rather than demonstrating that you have an understanding of the subject.

Remember that your aim at interview is to stand out from the crowd.

When answering this and similar questions, improvise your answer around a few subheadings.

Use of buzzwords/key phrases

To score maximum points with the interview panel it helps to mention certain buzzwords and key phrases in your answer. For example, with EBM you could talk about:

- Making use of *current best research evidence*
- Combining EBM with your *clinical expertise*
- Using EBM to make decisions about the *care of individual patients*
- Taking into account the *patients' values*

   To demonstrate your understanding further, think of an example of how you practise EBM.

Continued

Continued

> 'Evidence-based medicine is about making use of the *current best available research evidence* when making decisions about the care of *individual patients*. It involves combining *good evidence*, preferably category A or B, with one's own *clinical expertise*, taking into account the patients' *preferences, concerns and expectations*.
>
>   'I regularly make use of respected resources such as Medline and "Up-to-date" to conduct literature reviews and integrate this with my clinical practice taking into account my patients' views and seeking their feedback.'
>
>   This provides a much more effective answer than simply regurgitating a ready-made definition. Note that in this case, 'patient values' was substituted by 'patients' preferences, concerns and expectations', which helps to demonstrate that you understand what is meant by the term 'patient values'.

When you mention key phrases, such as 'clinical expertise', you should be prepared for subsequent questions to check your understanding of that phrase.

'What is meant by best available research evidence?'
This refers to clinically relevant research, especially patient-centred research, concerning:
- The accuracy and precision of diagnostic tests
- The power of prognostic markers
- The efficacy and safety of therapeutic, rehabilitative and preventative treatments.

'What is meant by clinical expertise?'
This refers to a clinician's ability to use their skills and past experience to identify a patient's:
- Health state and diagnosis
- Individual risk and benefit of potential interventions
- Personal values and expectations.

'What is meant by patient values?'
Each patient will bring unique preferences, concerns and expectations to a clinical encounter. These three elements must be integrated into clinical decisions for the patient's best interests.

> **Summary: how to practise EBM**
>
> - A clinical problem arises out of the care of a patient
> - A well-defined clinical question is constructed from the case
> - A search is conducted using the most appropriate resources
> - Evidence is appraised for its validity (i.e. closeness to the truth) and applicability (i.e. usefulness in clinical practice)
> - Evidence is integrated with clinical practice and patient preferences and application to practice
> - Performance is evaluated with the patient

'Can you give us an example of how you practise EBM?'

When answering this question, be specific. Consider, for your specialty, what clinical problems arise with your patients. For example:

- A patient presents with benign essential tremor
- Discussing treatment options with a patient with rheumatoid arthritis
- Discussing treatment options for Dukes B colorectal cancer

  Think about where you source your evidence, for example:

- On-line resources such as Medline, Up-to-date, Cochrane database
- Peer-reviewed journals such as the *British Medical Journal* (BMJ), the *Lancet* or the *New England Journal of Medicine* (NEJM)
- Institutions such as the National Institute for Health and Clinical Excellence (NICE)

  Think about how you appraise and integrate evidence:

- Does the evidence arise from a double-blind randomised control trial of suitable size?
- Has the research been criticised?
- Is it relevant to your clinical question and to your patient?

> **The different levels of evidence for EBM**
>
> Note the key phrases in *italics*:
>
> Level 1: Strong evidence from at least one published *systematic review* of multiple well-designed randomised controlled trials (RCTs).
>
> Level 2: Strong evidence from at least one *published appropriately designed RCT* of appropriate size and clinical setting.

Continued

Continued

Level 3: Evidence from published well-designed trials *without randomisation*, for example, single group pre–post, cohort, time series or matched case-controlled studies.

Level 4: Evidence from well-designed *non-experimental studies* from more than one centre or research group.

Level 5: *Opinions of respected authorities* based on clinical evidence, descriptive studies or reports of expert consensus committees.

These levels of evidence have been put into four commonly used categories:

Category A: Consistent level 1 studies.

Category B: Consistent level 2 or 3 studies, or extrapolations from level 1 studies.

Category C: Level 4 studies, or extrapolations from level 2 or 3 studies.

Category D: Level 5 evidence or inconclusive studies of any level.

'Do you think that EBM is applicable to all specialties?'

Here are some points to consider when answering this question:

- There may not be Category A evidence in the literature to address the clinical question, in which case clinicians should consider the next level of evidence. There may be no good evidence at all to support clinical judgement.
- Certain specialties benefit more than others due to research activity and clinical trials, for example Cardiology.
- There may not be a great body of evidence behind some older established treatments, which does not necessarily mean that they are not effective.

EBM on the web

- www.ebm.bmj.com
- www.theCochraneLibrary.com
- www.cebm.net

5.3 Audit and research

Questions about audit and research are very common at medical interviews. You need to be extremely familiar with your own audits and research. In addition, you need to have a good understanding of the principles of audit and research.

'What is audit?'

'Audit is the systematic, critical analysis of the quality of medical care, including the procedures used for diagnosis and treatment, to help to provide reassurance that the best quality of service is being achieved, having regard to the available resources.'

Alternatively, and described more simply: 'Audit is a peer review of health care to check on and improve services.'

If asked this question, you should answer it in a way that is more clinically relevant, by using an example of your own audits or your own clinical practice.

'What is the audit cycle?'

The audit cycle (Figure 5.1) first requires the setting of standards. This is followed by an observation of existing practice. A comparison is then made between the observed and set standards. Standards may be set locally or nationally. The National Service Frameworks (NSFs) and NICE provide a large number of standards for clinical practice.

Following comparison, some change should be carried out to improve existing practice. The final stage is to re-audit clinical practice at a specified future date following the implementation of change.

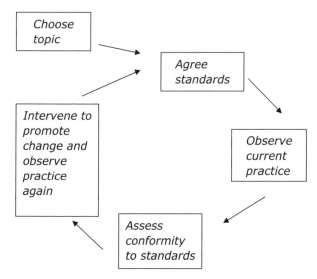

Figure 5.1 The audit cycle.

'Why is audit important?'

Audit is considered important for a number of reasons:

- The principal objective of audit is to improve the quality of service being provided
- Audit can lead to better use of resources and increased efficiency
- Audit can be a useful tool for training and education
- Audit can provide evidence to other institutions of the effectiveness of your service
- Audit is an important component in the implementation of clinical governance.

'Tell us about your audit experience'

It is important that you re-read all of your completed audits. For each of your audits, make a summary as described below. This summary should provide the basis for answering this question.

- Why did you choose the audit?
- How did you agree on the standards?
- How did you observe current practice and what were the main findings?
- What problems did you encounter?
- How did practice change as a result of your audit?
- What specifically was your role in the audit?

'What problems can arise with the audit process?'

Problems with audit can arise for a large number of reasons. With projects carried out by junior doctors, these are the principal causes:

- There is frequently a high turnover of junior doctors whose main focus is passing postgraduate exams. Consequently audits are often rushed, or thought of as a 'box-ticking' exercise for the CV. This leads to ill thought out or uncompleted audit projects
- Results are not presented and recommendations for change as a result of audit are not implemented
- The audit cycle may take some time to complete and is often not completed within the time framework available to a junior doctor.

'What is the difference between audit and research?'

This can be a scary question if you have not considered it prior to interview. It is particularly likely to be asked at higher ST grade interviews.

- Research is a systematic investigation, which aims to generate new knowledge and establish best practice
- Audit is a peer review of health care to check on/improve services.

The key differences between audit and research		
	Research	Audit
May involve an experimental approach	Yes	No
May involve a new treatment	Yes	No
Is applicable in other settings	Yes	No
Involves strict selection criteria for participant involvement	Yes	No
Usually conducted by those providing the service	No	Yes

'Can you think of an audit suitable for your practice?'

This is a good question designed to see if a candidate really considers the audit process as a useful tool. It is worth thinking of something that you would like to audit. It is important to demonstrate enthusiasm when answering! The answer will very much depend on your experience or chosen specialty. Examples could include:

- Vaccine uptake
- Appropriate antibiotic use and adherence to guidelines
- Adherence to asthma/MI/DKA guidelines

  These are some likely interview questions about research:

- 'Why is research important?'
- 'How has research affected your clinical practice?'
- 'What experience do you have of research?'
- 'What benefits have you gained from your research projects?'

5.4 Clinical governance

Questions that test a candidate's knowledge and understanding of clinical governance are common at medical interviews.

'Tell us about clinical governance'

The most widely used definition of clinical governance is this:

A framework through which NHS organizations are accountable for continually improving the quality of their services and safeguarding high standards of care by creating an environment in which excellence in clinical care will flourish.

Scally G, Donaldson LJ.

Don't try to memorise this definition. Instead, try to understand what is meant by this concept. Construct your own definition using the following buzzwords/key phrases:

- Framework
- Accountability
- Improving/maintaining standards of care
- Quality assurance process.

'Who is responsible for clinical governance?'

Within Hospitals, the responsibility for implementation belongs to the Chief Executive. (For that reason it is probably the Chief Executive asking the question.) Much of the implementation is delegated through the Medical Director, Clinical Directors, Consultants and other clinical staff. All doctors have a role to play in its implementation.

In primary care, responsibility lies with designated clinical governance leads.

The seven pillars of clinical governance

1. *Clinical effectiveness and research*
This relates to the use of effective treatments for patients and involves:
- Practising evidence-based medicine (see above)
- Implementing and supporting National Service Frameworks (NSFs) (see later)
- Being aware of local priorities for health care.

2. *Risk management*
This relates to having robust systems in place to learn from mistakes and to understand, monitor and minimise the risks to patients and staff. Risk management includes:
- The use of critical incident forms to report significant adverse events or 'near-miss' situations
- Identifying risks and assessing the probability of occurrence and the potential impact if an incident occurred
- Creating a 'blame-free culture' which encourages doctors and other clinical staff to feel safe about admitting mistakes.

3. *Education and training*
Professional development should continue through lifelong learning for all staff in order for them to keep up to date. For doctors this includes:
- Attending courses
- Appraisals
- On-the-job training.

Continued

Continued

4. *Patient and public involvement*

This relates to obtaining patient feedback and learning from their experiences. It is about putting the patient first. Institutions such as the National Patient Safety Agency (NPSA) and the Patient Advice Liaison Service (PALS) contribute to this process.

5. *Using information*

A large amount of confidential patient information is held by the NHS. To be able to access it efficiently and to protect confidentiality staff need to:

- Learn how to use computers
- Understand how the Data Protection Act relates to their work

The Caldicott Report, published in 1997, outlined the following principles aimed at improving medical confidentiality within the NHS:

- The use of patient data should be justified
- Patient identifiable information should only be used when absolutely necessary
- The minimum patient identifiable information should be used.
- Patient identifiable information should be accessed on a 'need to know' basis
- All staff should be aware of their responsibilities to maintain confidentiality
- There should be compliance with the Data Protection Act.

6. *Clinical audit*

See the section on audit above.

7. *Staffing and staff management*

The final pillar of clinical governance relates to staff recruitment, management and development. In addition, effective methods of working and good working conditions are incorporated.

With a good understanding of clinical governance you should be able to answer the following potential interview questions:

- 'In what way does clinical governance impact on your daily work?'
- 'Who is responsible for clinical governance in your workplace?'
- 'Do you think clinical governance is useful, or is it a waste of time?'
- 'What problems are there with the way clinical governance is implemented?'

Clinical governance on the web

- Clinical Governance Support Team: www.cgsupport.nhs.uk
- Department of Health: www.dh.gov.uk

5.5 The National Patient Safety Agency (NPSA)

Patients are seen as having an integral role in the current and future development of the NHS. Increasingly, lay members are invited to sit on interview panels. This is indeed becoming commonplace at interviews for more senior posts. Consequently, you might easily be asked about organisations that support patient involvement in the development of the NHS.

'What is the National Patient Safety Agency?'

The NPSA is a special Health Authority created in 2001 to co-ordinate the efforts of the entire country to report, and more importantly to learn from, mistakes and problems that affect patient safety. The role of the NPSA includes:

- Collecting incident reports from across the country and initiating preventative measures, so that the whole country can learn from each case
- Promoting an open and fair culture across the Health Service, encouraging all staff to report incidents and 'near-misses' without fear of reprimand with the emphasis more about the 'how' than the 'who'
- Safety aspects of hospital design
- Cleanliness and food
- Ensuring research is carried out safely, through its responsibility for the Central Office for Research Ethics Committees (COREC).

'Why was the NPSA created?'

It has been estimated that there are 900 000 incidents either harming or nearly harming NHS hospital in-patients in the UK each year. In 2000, an expert group led by Dr Liam Donaldson, Chief Medical Officer, produced a report called 'An organisation with a memory'. This report acknowledged that there had been little systematic learning from patient safety incidents and service failure in the NHS in the past and drew attention to the scale of the problem of potentially avoidable events that result in unintended harm to patients.

The report proposed the introduction of a new national system for identifying patient safety incidents to reduce risk and prevent similar events occurring in the future.

The National Patient Safety Agency website

- www.npsa.nhs.uk

5.6 Politics and the Health Service

No, don't move on to the next chapter!!!!

The rest of this chapter covers some important aspects around how the Health Service functions across the UK. It also covers crucial issues around evolving education and training for junior doctors as well as contracts for more senior doctors.

You will probably be asked about some current political issues affecting the Health Service and developments in training or job planning. We cannot tell which questions these will be. However, they are likely to cover issues that relate to your chosen career.

A common reason for failing at interview is because a candidate 'falls to pieces' after being asked a question that he/she did not understand. Typically, this may be as a result of hearing a political term or Health Service jargon. If you take the time to read through our summary of some political developments in the NHS you are less likely to be entirely flummoxed by a question that refers to 'Choose and book' or 'Practice-based commissioning'. This may give you the edge over other candidates.

Summary: a brief history of the National Health Service (NHS)

The NHS was set up in 1948 to provide health care for all citizens, based on need, rather than ability to pay. It was the brainchild of Aneurin Bevan, Minister for Health in the pioneering Labour government which swept into power after the Second World War.

The NHS is funded by the taxpayer and is managed by the Department of Health that sets overall policy on health issues.

Since 1948 there have been huge changes to both the organisational structure of the NHS and the way that patient services are provided. Some of the more important recent events are outlined below and discussed in more detail later in this chapter:

- *1991*: Creation of NHS Trusts and GP fund-holding allowing some family doctors to have budgets to 'buy' health care from NHS trusts
- *1997*: NICE (National Institute of Clinical Excellence; since renamed National Institute for Health and Clinical Excellence) agency established
- *1998*: Launch of NHS Direct, the nurse-led health advice service
- *1998*: NSFs (National Service Frameworks) established
- *2000*: NHS Plan published
- *2000*: Perhaps the most prolific serial killer in British history, Dr Harold Shipman, was convicted of 15 counts of murder

- *2002*: Creation of Primary Care Trusts (PCTs) as well as Strategic Health Authorities (SHAs), replacing the former Health Authorities, taking on a strategic role in improving local health services
- *2003*: Consultants in England voted in favour of a new contract
- *2004*: Introduction of the new General Medical Services (GMS) contract for GPs
- *2005*: Launch of Foundation programmes replacing the Pre-registration House Officer (PRHO) year as part of Modernising Medical Careers (MMC).
- *2007*: Launch of Specialist Training programmes replacing SHO and Registrar grades as part of MMC.

'What is the NHS Plan?'

Published in 2000, the NHS Plan was a 10-year plan for healthcare reform in the UK, promising increased funding for the NHS. The planned changes aimed to empower patients, by involving them in the referral process and giving them greater choice on where they get treatment. The plan required new common national standards and prices, as well as independent inspection throughout the NHS.

The NHS Plan promised:
- More information for patients
- More hospitals and beds
- More doctors and nurses
- Shorter waiting times
- Better hospital facilities
- Improved care for older people
- Higher standards for NHS organisations.

The NHS Plan prioritised certain key areas of health care, targeting diseases such as coronary heart disease and cancer. This aimed to specify the most urgent changes for the delivery of better healthcare services.

Much has happened since the NHS Plan was first published, but every development and initiative coming after has its roots in the NHS Plan's core vision of creating a patient-led NHS. The aim is that services are built on the needs and preferences of patients linking up all the services and care a patient requires. Wherever possible, it was stated that services and care should be offered in convenient community settings closer to the patient's home.

5.7 Organisation of health care in the UK

It is worthwhile having a basic understanding of the way that health care is organised and financed in the UK, especially for senior medical interviews.

Organisation of UK health care

- *Department of Health (DH)*: the DH plans the overall direction of the National Health Service, sets and monitors national healthcare standards.
- *Strategic Health Authorities (SHAs)*: regional management of the NHS is devolved to 28 SHAs, who monitor performance at a regional level and determine local strategy.
- *Special Health Authorities*: in addition to the regional SHAs, a number of Special Health Authorities provide specialist services across England. These include the National Blood Authority, which co-ordinates blood donations and distribution.
- *Primary care*: health care is divided into primary and secondary care. Primary care refers to the health services first visited by those who have a health problem. These are GPs, dentists, opticians, pharmacists, Walk-in health centres and NHS Direct.
- *Secondary care*: secondary care includes NHS Hospital Trusts, Mental Health Trusts, ambulance trusts and social care services. Patients who need care that cannot be provided by primary care will be referred to secondary care services by a primary care practitioner or will be taken directly to these services in an emergency.
- *Primary Care Trusts (PCTs)*: PCTs are responsible for the provision of health services to the local community. PCTs are allocated money from SHAs and they control 75% of the NHS budget. PCTs are responsible for the provision of primary care and the planning of secondary care with secondary care service providers.
- *NHS Trusts*: NHS Trusts are responsible for running many NHS hospitals. They are accountable to their regional SHA.
- *Mental Health Trusts:* Mental Health Trusts oversee mental health services which can be provided through a GP, other primary care services or through more specialist care in NHS Hospital Trusts or local council social services departments.

When you are asked about the medical and political systems or organisations described here, try to answer with examples where you have had personal contact or experience. This will sound impressive at interview.

'How is the NHS financed?'

After the chancellor collects tax, a proportion of his budget is allocated to the Department of Health (DH). The DH distributes this money to Strategic Health Authorities (SHAs) who in turn distribute it to Primary Care Trusts (PCTs). PCTs then commission (buy) services from NHS Hospitals, Foundation Hospitals, private Hospitals or Independent Service Treatment Centres (ISTCs).

'What is Practice-based commissioning?'

Practice-based commissioning (PBC) enables GP practices to:
- Operate as independent businesses with their own budgets
- Purchase the services they need from a variety of providers (NHS or private)
  Advocates of PBC believe that increased competition will lead to improved quality of services, greater patient choice and better care for patients.
  Some of the concerns/criticisms of PBC are that:
- This is NHS 'privatisation' via the back door
- GPs will refer fewer patients to save money
- GPs will refer patients to providers in which they have a financial interest
- Hospital managers should have greater say in the type of services available.

PBC on the web

- www.primarycarecontracting.nhs.uk

'What is "Choose and book"?'

Choose and book (CAB) is an electronic booking service that was introduced in 2006. It gives patients the opportunity to choose a secondary care appointment at a convenient time and location. CAB works as follows:
- The patient receives an appointment request letter from their GP, with a reference number and password and a list of hospitals/clinics, that have been commissioned by the PCT, to choose from
- Patients are given information on hospital facilities such as car parking, as well as performance ratings
- Patients can book their appointment either through the CAB telephone line or website, by calling the clinic directly or through their GP surgery
- The specialist will be able to access the referral letter beforehand and, depending on the appropriateness of the referral, can alter the priority status, or reject the referral, in which case the GP is notified.
  Advantages of CAB include:
- Better flexibility and choice for patients
- The referral letter getting to the specialist electronically and in good time
- A reduction in 'Did Not Attend' (DNA) patients
  Disadvantages of CAB include:
- A system that is confusing for vulnerable patients such as the elderly
- Patients will only be offered services commissioned by the PCT, meaning that some clinics could be forced to close down
- Discussing possible options means that GP consultation times increase.

'What are Private Finance Initiatives?'

Private Finance Initiatives (PFIs) provide a way of funding major capital investments, for example hospitals, without immediate recourse to the public purse. Private consortia, usually involving large construction firms, are contracted to design, build and in some cases manage new projects. Contracts typically last for 30 years, during which time a public authority, such as an NHS Trust, leases the building.

'What are the advantages and disadvantages of single-handed GP practices?'

Since the Shipman inquiry, GPs have been encouraged to move away from single-handed practices towards 'super-practices', so that doctors work under closer scrutiny.

Advantages of 'super-practices' include:
- Uniting a number of GPs with special interests
- Better opportunities for GPs to keep up to date
- Ability to offer a wide range of services to patients
  Disadvantages of 'super-practices' include:
- Patients may end up seeing different doctors and not get such good continuation of care
- Patients may have to travel further to the nearest practice
- They are less suited to rural areas.

'What are Independent Service Treatment Centres (ISTCs)?'

ISTCs are treatment centres run by private companies. PCTs can commission ISTCs to perform a certain number of treatments, perhaps 500 hernia operations. Their aim is to reduce waiting times without taking staff away from existing local NHS services.

ISTCs have been criticised for not offering good aftercare as well as affecting training for junior doctors by taking away routine cases.

'What is a Foundation Hospital/Trust?'

NHS Foundation Trusts are part of government strategy aiming to decentralise public services.

If a hospital is seen as performing well, it can apply for Foundation status. The aim of Foundation Trusts is to devolve decision making from central government control to local organisations and communities so they are more responsive to the needs and wishes of their local people.

This means that Trusts have greater autonomy and can borrow money, buy or sell land, and offer performance-related salaries to staff. The hospital's income is related to its performance.

5.8 The Healthcare Commission

'What is the Healthcare Commission?'

The Healthcare Commission is an independent body, set up to promote and drive improvement in the quality of health care and public health. Its legal name is the 'Commission for Healthcare Audit and Inspection'. It replaced the 'Commission for Health Improvement' (CHI) in 2004 and is a healthcare watchdog.

'What does the Healthcare Commission do?'

In England, the role of the Healthcare Commission includes:

- Inspecting the quality and value for money of health care and public health
- Reviewing the performance of each NHS Trust and awarding an annual performance rating
- Supplying patients and the public with the best possible information about the provision of health care
- Promoting improvements in health care and public health
- Regulating the independent healthcare sector
- Investigating serious failures in the provision of health care.

'What about Scotland and Wales?'

The Healthcare Commission does not cover Scotland as it has its own body, NHS Quality Improvement Scotland.

Local inspection and investigation of NHS bodies in Wales rests with the Healthcare Inspectorate Wales.

The annual 'health check'

In April 2005 the Healthcare Commission launched a new approach to assessing and rating the performance of each local NHS organisation: the annual 'health check'.

Replacing the old system of 'star ratings', its stated aim is to promote improvements in health care for patients and the public, looking at a broad range of issues such as:

- Whether organisations are meeting 24 core standards of care—these set out the basic level of care that Trusts should be providing
- How well they manage their finances and other resources
- The findings from individual reviews, which focus on specific areas of health care such as services for children and diagnostics

---

Continued

Continued

> Each year the Healthcare Commission publishes an annual performance rating for each organisation which has two parts:
> **1.** Quality of services
> **2.** Use of resources
>   The ratings are published on a four-point scale: excellent, good, fair or weak, and are published on the Healthcare Commission website.

Top tip: we would strongly recommend that you familiarise yourself with the relevant Healthcare Commission's annual health check for the Trust to which you are applying, especially for senior medical interviews.

Healthcare inspection on the web

- Healthcare Commission: www.healthcarecommission.org.uk
- NHS Quality Improvement Scotland: www.nhshealthquality.org
- Health Inspectorate Wales: www.hiw.org.uk

5.9 Consultant and GP contracts

Both Consultant and GP contracts have recently been renegotiated. We have summarised the key features that you need to be aware of if you are asked about these topics at a medical interview.

The Consultant contract

The 2003 Consultant contract was negotiated between the BMA and the Department of Health. Most existing Consultants and all new Consultants working within the NHS from that date work according to that contract.

The new contract changed the measure of Consultants' work, and attaches a time value to programmed activities (PAs).

Attaching a time value to PAs is intended to provide greater transparency about the level of commitment expected of Consultants by the NHS.

The framework for full-time Consultants is 10 PAs each of 4 hours (3 hours at night), although many still find themselves working more.

The contract sets out that a full-time Consultant will typically devote on average of 7.5 programmed activities per week to Direct Clinical Care (DCC). DCC includes activity that involves the care of individual patients (such as clinic letters, multidisciplinary team meetings, seeing relatives, reviewing results, etc.)

Supporting professional activities (SPAs), additional NHS responsibilities and external duties are expected to contribute 2.5 PAs.

The precise balance is agreed as part of job plan reviews and may vary to take account of individual circumstances.

Important SPAs such as audit, teaching, research, appraisal, continuing professional development, clinical governance and service development may frequently take more than 2.5 sessions. This may well be a source of contention between Consultants and individual Trusts, and also between Royal Colleges and the Department of Health. There is also the additional role of educational supervision of doctors in training.

Predictable emergency work out-of-hours (such as ward rounds at evenings and weekends) is programmed into the working week.

Those with a major and regular commitment to undergraduate or postgraduate teaching should have that recognised within their job plan. A different version of the new Consultant contract for clinical academics has now been negotiated for Academic Consultants, who should have an integrated job plan agreed with their NHS Trust and University employers.

'What is the General Medical Services (GMS) contract?'
It is essential to have a good understanding of the GMS contract if you are applying for a post in General Practice.

The original GMS contract came into place in 2004 and was revised in 2006. It has been designed to reward GPs offering a wider range of services and a high standard of care. Some of the key elements of the contract are as follows:

Service categorisation
Under the GMS contract, practice services are categorised as follows:
- *Essential*: services that a practice must provide, for example management of ill patients, terminal care and chronic disease management
- *Additional*: services that practices are expected to provide, such as contraceptive services, but can opt out of
- *Enhanced*: services that the PCT can commission from practices reflecting patient need, for example specialist sexual health services.

Payment
PCTs allocate money to GP practices in three main ways:
- A *global sum* to cover essential and additional service provision
- *Enhanced* service payments
- *Quality payments* rewarding achieving quality standards.

If practices opt out of additional services, or out-of-hours services, they will have their global sum allocation reduced.

Quality and outcomes framework

Practices are assessed and awarded points (known as QOF points) which are converted to quality payments based on their performance in four areas with key indicators/defined quality standards:
- *Clinical*: e.g. care of diabetes, ischaemic heart disease
- *Organisational*: e.g. practice management
- *Patient experience*: e.g. use of patient questionnaires
- *Additional services*: e.g. undertaking cervical screening.

Information management and technology

PCTs will fund all of the IT systems needed to implement the contract.

Option to opt out of out-of-hours (OOH)

GP practices can opt out of OOH services (weekends and nights). Practices receive a reduced global sum payment and the PCT becomes responsible for arranging alternative provision.

The advantages for GPs in opting out of OOH are less stress and tiredness and a better work–life balance.

The disadvantages are that GPs are at risk of losing their acute skills, private providers may deliver a reduced quality of care and continuity of care may be lost.

GPs with special interests

Under the GMS contract, GPs with special interests (GPwSI, often referred to as 'Gypsies') can provide specialist services to patients. This can be more convenient for patients if the services are provided in a primary care setting, and can relieve the pressure on secondary care.

There are concerns that GPs may not be able to offer the same standard of care as a specialist, and that GPs with heavy specialist commitments might become deskilled in general practice.

5.10 Modernising Medical Careers (MMC)

'What is MMC?'

MMC became operational in 2005 and is a major reform of postgraduate education. Its aims are to improve patient care by delivering a modernised, focused career structure for doctors. The Pre-registration House Officer (PRHO),

Senior House Officer (SHO) and Registrar grades have been phased out and replaced by a new training structure for junior doctors.

'How did MMC come about?'

The events that led to the creation of MMC included:

- The NHS Plan which contained a commitment to modernise SHO training
- A report published by the Chief Medical Officer in 2002 called 'Unfinished business—proposals for reform of the senior house officer grade' highlighted problems including inadequate supervision, assessment, appraisal and career advice, with no defined end-point to training
- With the implementation of the European Working Time Directive (EWTD), and reduced working hours, it was felt that a more structured training was needed.

MMC was the response of UK Health Ministers to these events. They agreed the introduction of the Foundation programme, and the establishment of a run-through training grade — amalgamating the current SHO and specialist Registrar grades into Specialist Training (ST) posts.

'What are Foundation programmes?'

Foundation years one (F1) and two (F2) make up the 2-year Foundation programme, which has replaced the PRHO year and the first year of SHO training. Some key features of Foundation programmes include:

- All UK medical graduates are required to undertake the Foundation programme before progressing to specialty or GP training
- Foundation doctors are trained and assessed against specific competences set out in the Curriculum for the Foundation Years in Postgraduate Education and Training
- The F1 curriculum is based on GMC requirements and developing awareness of the important duties of doctors
- The F2 curriculum includes developing skills in handling common emergencies
- The GMC and the Postgraduate Medical Education and Training Board (PMETB) are responsible for the approval and quality assurance of the Foundation programme
- Deaneries are responsible for implementing and managing the programmes through Foundation Schools
- Foundation Schools bring together Medical Schools, postgraduate Deaneries and healthcare providers to provide training in a variety of specialties and settings.

'How does ST and GP run-through training work?'

A doctor can compete for a place on a run-through training programme to begin immediately upon successful completion of the Foundation programme. Some key features of training programmes include:

- Each programme has a curriculum, agreed by the PMETB, against which doctors in training will be assessed. The number of years that a trainee spends in training varies between programmes
- Doctors in Specialist or GP training have the opportunity to gain a Certificate of Completion of Training (CCT), subject to satisfactory progress
- After a doctor receives a CCT, they are legally eligible for entry to the Specialist or GP Register and can then apply for an appropriate senior medical appointment.

Fixed-term Specialist Training appointments (FTSTAs)

These appointments are for a fixed period of 1 year. They are designed to mirror the early years of training in a Specialty/GP training programme. They are educationally approved training posts that are under the auspices of the postgraduate Medical Dean. They are only available in hospital settings for the first 2 years after completion of Foundation posts.

Senior medical appointments

These cover GP principals, Consultants and other specialist roles. These roles are determined by the service.

Career posts

These positions are service delivery posts with no formal ST elements. However, employer appraisal and continuing professional development remain an essential component. They are only available in Hospital settings.

'What criticisms have been made of MMC?'

The new changes have not proceeded without criticism. Some of the concerns expressed and counter arguments are as follows:

- With MMC and the EWTD, the training time of doctors will be reduced, and there are concerns that Specialists will not have gained the necessary experience. It is hoped that a more efficient and structured training will offset this
- Trainees will have to decide on their chosen specialty after less than 2 years' postgraduate experience. This may lead to doctors making inappropriate career choices. Short 'tasters' are available to help doctors make their choices, and career advice is available
- Because the emphasis is on competencies acquired rather than experience gained, it is difficult to get work undertaken abroad recognised.

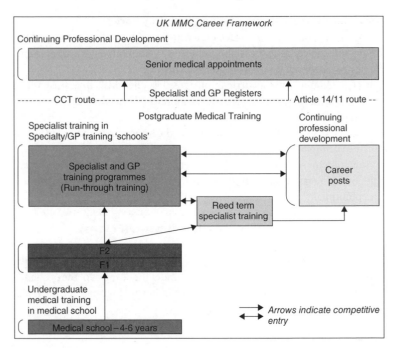

Figure 5.2 UK MMC career framework.

MMC on the web

- Official MMC website: www.mmc.nhs.uk
- MMC 360°: www.mmc360.com
- Remedy UK: www.remedyuk.org
- NHS Careers: www.nhscareers.nhs.uk

5.11 The European Working Time Directive (EWTD)

'What is the EWTD?'

The EWTD is a directive from the European Union to protect the health and safety of workers in the European Union. It lays down minimum requirements in relation to working hours, rest periods, annual leave and working arrangements for night workers. It was enacted in UK law in 1998, but doctors in training were exempt until 2004, at which time the directive was phased in with a maximum weekly working hours requirement reducing from 58 hours in 2004 to 48 hours in 2009.

'What are the key features of the EWTD?'

The important features of EWTD for workers are that there should be:

- No more than 48 hours' work per week (averaged over a reference period)
- 11 hours continuous rest in each 24 hour period
- 24 hours continuous rest in each 7 day period (or 48 hours in 14 days)
- 20 minute breaks in work periods of over 6 hours
- 4 weeks annual leave
- For night workers an average of no more than 8 hours' work in each 24 hour period.

'What is the SiMAP judgement?'

The SiMAP judgement refers to a case brought before the European Court of Justice on behalf of a group of Spanish doctors. The ruling declared that all time spent resident on-call would count as working time. While this ruling applied to a specific case, it is assumed that if British doctors work under similar arrangements, then a similar interpretation of 'working time' applies.

'Are GPs covered by the EWTD?'

No. GPs do not typically fall within the remit of the EWTD as they are often self-employed.

'What have been the consequences of the implementation of the EWTD?'

The introduction of the EWTD has had a profound effect on doctors' working patterns. There has been criticism that shift patterns of work have significantly impacted on the continuity of patient care. The EWTD has challenged the government to look at the way training is delivered, and it has been a contributing factor to the development of its MMC strategy (see earlier).

In order to achieve compliance with the EWTD, the government was forced to develop other strategies which have included:

- Hospital at Night (see below)
- Expansion of extended nursing roles
- Making more use of non-medical staff to support doctors.

5.12 Hospital at Night

'What is Hospital at Night?'

The Hospital at Night project aims to redefine how medical cover is provided in hospitals during the out-of-hours period in response to the EWTD. The Department of Health, the NHS Modernisation Agency, the BMA and the Royal Colleges are all stakeholders in Hospital at Night.

The key elements of Hospital at Night include:
- Working in multidisciplinary teams
- Multispecialist handovers
- Bleep filtering
- Extended nursing roles
- Moving non-urgent work from the night-time.

EWTD and Hospital at Night on the web

- www.healthcareworkforce.nhs.uk

5.13　General Medical Council

'What is the role of the GMC?'

All practising medical doctors in the UK must be registered with the GMC. It has legal powers to protect, promote and maintain the health and safety of the public by ensuring proper standards in the practice of medicine.

The GMC legally has four main functions under the Medical Act:
- Keeping up-to-date registers of qualified doctors
- Fostering good medical practice
- Promoting high standards of medical education
- Dealing firmly and fairly with doctors whose fitness to practise is in doubt.

The GMC has been criticised in the past for being overly protective of doctors, particularly following the Shipman inquiry. The GMC was forced to undergo reform, which had three main elements:
- Reducing the size of the council and increasing the percentage of lay people on the council
- Reforming fitness to practise procedures
- Reforming doctors' registration procedures and introducing revalidation (working with the Department of Health).

A recent government white paper on medical regulation is 'Trust, assurance and safety—the regulation of Health Professionals in the 21st century'. It proposes improving medical standards through increased regulation.

The GMC website

- www.gmc-uk.org

5.14 Council for Healthcare Regulatory Excellence (CHRE)

'What is the CHRE?'

The CHRE is a statutory body, separate from the Department of Health, established in 2003. Its aims are to promote best practice and consistency in the regulation of healthcare professionals. The CHRE has the power to refer fitness to practise decisions made by the regulators to the High Court if it considers that the regulator's decision was 'unduly lenient'. It promotes best practice and consistency in the regulation of healthcare professionals by the following nine regulatory bodies:

- General Chiropractic Council
- General Dental Council
- General Medical Council
- General Optical Council
- General Osteopathic Council
- Health Professions Council
- Nursing and Midwifery Council
- Pharmaceutical Society of Northern Ireland
- Royal Pharmaceutical Society of Great Britain.

The CHRE website

- www.chre.org.uk

5.15 Postgraduate Medical Education and Training Board (PMETB)

'What is the PMETB?'

The PMETB is the independent statutory body responsible for postgraduate medical education and training for all specialties, including General Practice, across the UK.

The PMETB took over the responsibilities of the Specialist Training Authority of the Medical Royal Colleges and the Joint Committee on Postgraduate Training for General Practice in 2005.

The PMETB's responsibilities include:

- Certifying doctors for GP and ST posts
- Approving training posts for CCT (Certificate for Completion of Training)
- Approving curricula and assessments from medical Royal Colleges
- Quality assurance of training.

The PMETB website

• www.pmetb.org.uk

'What is the role of the Royal Colleges?'

There are Royal Colleges for all specialties. The role of individual colleges and faculties is to develop and advise the PMETB regarding the curriculum for each specialty, or subspecialty.

In advising and supporting the PMETB they:

- Publish curricula that identify the standards and competencies required for each specialty
- Recommend to the PMETB the awarding or withholding of educational approval posts, placements and programmes
- Determine the standards of professional education and training through examinations/assessments that trainees must pass
- Support the delivery of training programmes through regular inspection of approved posts, placement and programmes.

Top tip: familiarise yourself with the website of the relevant Royal College for your specialty.

Royal College websites

- Joint Royal Colleges of Physicians Training Board: www.jrcptb.org.uk
- Joint Committee on Higher Surgical Training: www.jchst.org
- Faculty of Occupational Medicine: www.facoccmed.ac.uk
- The College of Emergency Medicine: www.emergencymed.org.uk
- Faculty of Pharmaceutical Medicine: www.fpm.org.uk
- Faculty of Public Health: www.fph.org.uk
- Royal College of Anaesthetists: www.rcoa.org.uk
- Royal College of General Practitioners: www.rcgp.org.uk
- Royal College of Obstetricians and Gynaecologists: www.rcog.org.uk
- Royal College of Ophthalmologists: www.rcophth.ac.uk
- Royal College of Paediatrics and Child Health: www.rcpch.ac.uk
- Royal College of Pathologists: www.rcpath.org
- Royal College of Physicians: www.rcplondon.ac.uk
- Royal College of Physicians and Surgeons of Glasgow: www.rcpsg.ac.uk
- Royal College of Surgeons of Edinburgh: www.rcsed.ac.uk
- Royal College of Physicians of Edinburgh: www.rcpe.ac.uk
- Royal College of Psychiatrists: www.rcpsych.ac.uk
- Royal College of Radiologists: www.rcr.ac.uk
- Royal College of Surgeons of England: www.rcseng.ac.uk

'What is the role of the Deanery?'

Deaneries have responsibility for postgraduate medical and dental education and training. Deaneries commission postgraduate medical and dental education, to standards set by the General Medical and Dental Councils and the PMETB. The Deanery's role includes:

- Contributing to workforce planning
- Maintaining a database of doctors and dentists in training
- Ensuring equality of opportunity in recruitment and progress through training programmes
- Ensuring that the performance and progress of all doctors and dentists in training are regularly, reliably and fairly assessed and recorded
- Providing careers information and advice
- Facilitating training for those with special needs
- Operational responsibility for ensuring that the Foundation programme is delivered to national standards set by the GMC and the PMETB.

Top tip: familiarise yourself with the relevant Deanery website before your interview (and preferably before you apply for the job!).

Deanery websites

- NHS Education for Scotland: www.nes.scot.nhs.uk
- Northern Deanery: mypimd.ncl.ac.uk
- North Western Deanery: www.pgmd.man.ac.uk
- Yorkshire Deanery: www.yorkshiredeanery.com
- South Yorkshire and South Humber Deanery: www.syshdeanery.com
- Mersey Deanery: www.merseydeanery.nhs.uk
- Trent Deanery: www.trentdeanery.nottingham.ac.uk
- West Midlands Deanery: www.wmdeanery.org
- Leicestershire, Northamptonshire and Rutland Deanery: www.lnrhwd.nhs.uk
- Eastern Deanery: www.easterndeanery.org
- Oxford Deanery: www.oxford-pgmde.co.uk
- London Deanery: www.londondeanery.ac.uk
- Kent, Surrey and Sussex Deanery: kssdeanery.ac.uk
- Severn Institute: www.severninstitute.nhs.uk
- Wessex Institute: www.wessexinstitute.nhs.uk
- South West Peninsula Deanery: www.peninsuladeanery.nhs.uk

5.16 National Institute for Health and Clinical Excellence (NICE)

'What is NICE?'

Established by the new Labour Government in 1997, NICE is an agency of the NHS which aims to drive up clinical standards in the NHS by developing guidance and recommendations on the effectiveness of treatments and medical procedures, and to ensure that improvements are consistent across the Health Service.

Prior to NICE, medical technology appraisals were carried out by a variety of professional and academic bodies, at both the national and local levels. Work was duplicated, standards were variable and the status of findings was frequently unclear.

'What does NICE do?'

NICE guidance is developed using the expertise of the NHS and the wider healthcare community including NHS staff, healthcare professionals, patients and carers, industry and the academic world.

NICE produces guidance in three areas of health:

- Public health — guidance on the promotion of good health
- Health technologies — guidance on the use of new and existing medicines, treatments and procedures
- Clinical practice — guidance on the appropriate treatment and care of people with specific diseases and conditions.

'What criticisms have been made of NICE?'

NICE has been highly controversial during its short lifetime, and has been criticised on a number of grounds. It is widely acknowledged that many of NICE's appraisals have been successful, and have improved standards in the NHS. At the heart of criticism directed towards NICE is the requirement that its decisions reflect the cost-effectiveness of treatments. This, it is argued, means that its clinical recommendations are inextricably tied up with political decisions relating to cost.

NICE is never far from the headlines. Two examples of controversy include:

- In June 2000 the credibility of NICE was challenged by its shift of position over the extremely expensive and clinically controversial multiple sclerosis drug beta interferon, primarily in response to patient pressure
- In June 2007 NICE published interim guidance on anti-VEGF treatments in ARMD restricting their use to second eyes (visual acuity worse than 6/9, classic subfoveal types only). This was controversial since anti-VEGF

treatments have been shown to be effective in almost all types of wet ARMD.

'Tell us about a NICE guideline that relates to your specialty'

This is a common interview question. You should be well prepared for it!

> **The NICE website**
>
> • www.nice.org.uk

5.17 National Service Frameworks

'What are NSFs?'

Launched in 1998 by the Department of Health as part of the Government's modernisation strategy, NSFs are long-term strategies for improving some of the highest priority conditions such as the UK's biggest killers, cancer and coronary heart disease, as well as other common conditions including mental health disorders and diabetes. There are also NSFs for key patient groups including children and older people.

NSFs have two main roles. They:
• Set clear quality requirements for care based on the best available evidence of what treatments and services work most effectively for patients
• Offer strategies and support to help organisations achieve these.

NSFs are developed by groups that include health professionals, service users and carers, health service managers, partner agencies, and other advocates.

'Tell me about an NSF relating to your specialty'

If your chosen specialty has an NSF that is relevant to it, this question will frequently be asked.

> **National Service Frameworks on the web**
>
> • www.dh.gov.uk/en/Policyandguidance/Healthandsocialcaretopics

5.18 Appraisal

You need to have a good understanding of appraisal, assessment and revalidation for an interview. You should bring documentary evidence of appraisals and assessments along with you to your interview.

'What is appraisal?'

Appraisal is a formal structured process for ensuring personal and professional development. Doctors should have regular formal meetings with their appraiser to reflect on their performance and identify development needs. It is neither an examination nor an assessment. Consultant educational or clinical supervisors commonly perform appraisals.

The aims of appraisal include:

- Reviewing work performance including contribution to education, research and to improving the quality of local healthcare services
- Constructing a Personal Development Plan (PDP) specifying personal and professional development needs, career path and goals, and agreeing methods to help achieve them
- Using the appraisal process and associated documentation to meet requirements for revalidation.

'How should doctors prepare for an appraisal?'

There is a standardised format for an appraisal. Doctors should prepare an appraisal folder that includes documentation of the personal development work done throughout the year. A large part of this may be collecting information on work that they are already carrying out, such as audits being performed or the journal articles that they have read.

'Who is responsible for appraisal of GPs?'

PCTs are responsible for the appraisal of GPs. They must ensure that appraisers are trained and can appraise the whole scope of a doctor's duties including clinical performance and, where appropriate, service delivery and management. Appraisals for GPs are based on the seven headings set out in *Good Medical Practice (2006)* available at the GMC website www.gmc-uk.org.

Appraisal on the web

- NHS Appraisal for Doctors Group: www.appraisalsupport.nhs.uk
- Department of Health: www.dh.gov.uk

5.19 Assessment

'What is assessment and how does it differ from appraisal?'

Assessment is a process to measure progress against defined criteria based on relevant curricula, whereas appraisal is a complementary process focusing on the trainee for ensuring personal and professional development. An appraisal is not a test.

'What is the difference between competence assessment and performance assessment?'

Competence assessment measures a practitioner's abilities under controlled circumstances, whereas performance assessment is a measure of ability and performance at work. Performance is not necessarily predicted by competence assessment and is thought to be more authentic since it assesses how a doctor performs during the working day with its inherent stresses and distractions.

Different types of assessment have been developed and incorporated into MMC. They are used to assess a doctor's competence.

When answering questions about assessment and appraisal, try wherever possible to use answers that relate to your own experience rather than using standardised textbook replies.

Summary: different types of assessment

MultiSource Feedback (MSF)

Mini-Peer Assessment Tool (Mini-PAT) and Team Assessment Behaviour (TAB) are MSF tools used to collate views from a range of co-workers for 360° assessment. The trainee nominates assessors to fill out a questionnaire. The trainee and educational supervisor agree strengths and key areas for development from the collated feedback.

Clinical evaluation exercise (Mini-CEX)

Mini-CEX is a 15-minute snapshot of doctor–patient interaction. It is designed to assess the clinical skills, attitudes and behaviour of trainees. Immediate feedback is provided after each encounter by the observer rating the trainee. Trainers and trainees identify agreed strengths, areas for development and an action plan for each encounter.

Direct Observation of Procedural Skills (DOPS)

DOPS are designed to provide feedback on procedural skills essential to the provision of good clinical care. Trainees undertake observed encounters, with different observers for each encounter. The trainee chooses the timing, procedure and observer.

Case-based Discussion (CbD)

The trainee selects case records from patients they have recently seen and in whose notes they have made an entry. The discussion starts from, and is centred upon, the trainee's record in the notes and is designed to assess the trainee's clinical decision making and their application or use of medical knowledge. It enables discussion of the ethical and legal framework of practice, and it allows trainees to discuss why they acted as they did.

Continued

Continued

Record of In-Training Assessment (RITA)

The RITA is an annual review process. It is not an assessment in itself but the assessment will have been ongoing and carried out by the educational supervisor (and colleagues) throughout a training placement.

Assessment on the web

- MMC: www.mmc.nhs.uk/pages/assessment
- Healthcare Assessment and Training: www.hcat.nhs.uk

5.20 Revalidation

'What is revalidation?'

Revalidation is a process by which doctors are assessed to ensure they remain up to date and fit to practise. All doctors are expected to maintain a folder of information about their practice. Every 5 years doctors will have to prove that they are fit to practise Medicine in order to renew their licence.

'Why has revalidation been drawn up?'

The GMC came under great pressure to reform doctor regulation in the wake of the Bristol Babies and Alder Hey Organ scandals. After GP Harold Shipman was convicted of murder in 2000, the government warned the GMC to develop tough self-regulation or it would impose it. Since then there have been several revalidation pilot schemes. For up-to-date information on revalidation, you should look at the suggested weblinks:

Revalidation on the web

- GMC: www.gmc-uk.org/doctors/licensing
- Department of Health: www.dh.gov.uk

'How does appraisal relate to revalidation?'

The differences between appraisal and revalidation are listed below:

Appraisal	Revalidation
Annual	Every 5 years
Developmental	An assessment
Aim is personal and professional development	Necessary for renewal of licence
Undertaken by trained appraiser	Undertaken by revalidation group

5.21 Summary

- Read through this entire chapter so that you have some understanding of important and topical changes relevant to your career. This might stop you from freezing during your interview
- Try to have a good understanding of the topics most relevant to your specialty
- Develop your own opinions about subjects and think how they relate to your work and the job you are applying for
- When expressing your opinions, be sure to keep them balanced and non-controversial. Remember that you do not know the views of each panel member
- Avoid textbook definitions whenever possible. Always try to give answers that relate to your own practice or experience
- Keep up to date with latest developments. The internet is a fantastic tool for helping you do this.

References

Sackett DL, Rosenberg WM, Gray JAM, *et al*. Evidence based medicine: what it is and what it isn't. *BMJ* 1996; **312**: 71–72

Sackett DL, Rosenberg W, Haynes BR. *Evidence-Based Medicine: How to Practice and Teach Evidence-Based Medicine*. New York: Churchill Livingstone, 2000

Scally G, Donaldson LJ. Clinical governance and the drive for quality improvement in the new NHS in England. *BMJ* 1998; **317**: 61–65.

Chapter 6 Interview questions that test your generic skills

6.1 Introduction

The aim of this chapter is to help you demonstrate your understanding and application of generic skills at interview. In order to do this, you need to understand what generic skills are and how they are tested at interview.

These questions can reveal a lot about a candidate and are liked by interviewers. They are frequently asked at both GP and ST interviews.

What are generic skills?

Generic (meaning general) skills are skills that are useable in a variety of contexts. They are core skills, or competencies, that are considered important for doctors.

Rather than specific skills, such as competency with a surgical technique or coronary angiography, generic skills are less specific. Examples of generic skills include communication, teamwork and organisation.

In order to understand and develop a good set of generic skills, it is important to be familiar with 'The duties of a doctor registered with the General Medical Council' (see later). It also helps to have a good knowledge and understanding of ethical and legal issues in health care. This includes an understanding of terms such as autonomy, beneficence, non-malfeasance, justice, capacity, consent, and issues that relate to confidentiality. These terms are explained later.

How are generic skills tested?

Generic skills can be tested in different ways such as:
- Being asked about your understanding of a specific term (such as 'empathy' or 'Gillick competence'). It is therefore important to have a good

How to Succeed at the Medical Interview By C. Smith and D. Meeking. 2008 by Blackwell Publishing, ISBN: 978-1-4051-6729-1.

understanding of a range of these terms and to work out your own personal definitions
- Being asked to give an example that highlights your use of generic skills, for example, 'Tell me about a time when you had to negotiate with a colleague'
- Being given a scenario that is relevant to a generic skill, for example, 'What would you do if you suspected that your colleague was drinking alcohol at work?'
- Being asked to participate in a role-play or patient simulation exercise
- Being asked to take part in a group discussion
- Performing a problem-solving exercise.

The final three examples will be discussed in detail in Chapter 7.

6.2 Understanding generic skills

When preparing how best to answer questions that test your understanding of generic skills it is essential to familiarise yourself with 'The duties of a doctor registered with the General Medical Council'. This is taken from *Good Medical Practice (2006)* and can be viewed on the GMC website www.gmc-uk.org.

The duties of a doctor registered with the General Medical Council

Patients must be able to trust doctors with their lives and health. To justify that trust you must show respect for human life and you must:
- Make the care of your patient your first concern
- Protect and promote the health of patients and the public
- Provide a good standard of practice and care
    - Keep your professional knowledge and skills up to date
    - Recognise and work within the limits of your competence
    - Work with colleagues in the ways that best serve patients' interests
- Treat patients as individuals and respect their dignity
    - Treat patients politely and considerately
    - Respect patients' right to confidentiality
- Work in partnership with patients
    - Listen to patients and respond to their concerns and preferences
    - Give patients the information they want or need in a way they can understand

---

Continued

Continued

> – Respect patients' right to reach decisions with you about their treatment and care
> – Support patients in caring for themselves to improve and maintain their health
> • Be honest and open and act with integrity
> – Act without delay if you have good reason to believe that you or a colleague may be putting patients at risk
> – Never discriminate unfairly against patients or colleagues
> – Never abuse your patients' trust in you or the public's trust in the profession
> You are personally accountable for your professional practice and must always be prepared to justify your decisions and actions.
>
> (Taken from the GMC website: www.gmc-uk.org)

Your knowledge and understanding of a doctor's duties could be assessed in an interview situation in the following ways:

- You may be asked how you keep your professional knowledge and skills up to date
- You may be given a patient simulation exercise where your communication skills are assessed
- You may be given a scenario where you have good reason to believe that a colleague of yours is not fit to practise.

The four ethical principles

You should be aware of the four largely accepted ethical principles that guide medical practice:

- *Autonomy*: this relates to a patient's individual dignity, and is about respect for the individual and their ability to make decisions with regard to their own health and future. Actions that enhance autonomy are thought of as desirable and actions that 'dwarf' an individual and their autonomy are considered to be undesirable.
- *Beneficence*: Patients visit doctors because of the expectation that the doctor can provide some good or relief. This relates to doing the greatest good whilst balancing risks and benefits. Doctors have an obligation to benefit the patient.
- *Non-malfeasance*: This relates to minimising harm. Doctors must avoid causing harm and strive to protect the patient from harm.
- *Justice*: This relates to fairness, equitable use of resources and equal access to care. Individuals or groups should be similarly treated and there should be

awareness that an individual's treatment may affect the well-being of someone else as a consequence of scarce resources.

These four principles can be thought of as guidelines to help you focus on ethical problems. Finding a solution to an ethical dilemma requires a consideration of each of these principles. It may not be clear which principles are more important. Interviewers like to explore these difficult ethical areas in order to learn more about candidates. Here are some examples of typical interview topics for you to consider:

- Balancing the patient's wishes to make decisions about their health care against the patient's wishes for doctor-assisted suicide.
- Balancing beneficence for an unborn child against respecting the autonomy of a woman who wants to terminate her pregnancy.
- Weighing up beneficence and justice owed to one person against another. How do we decide to whom we donate an organ?

In an interview situation you will be assessed on your knowledge and understanding of ethical principles and the thought process you use to guide your decisions. Your actual conclusion is less important as there is rarely a right or wrong answer; it is more important that you understand the issues involved. And remember at all times that each member of the interview panel will have their own opinions. Avoid being judgemental and provide a balanced response to difficult ethical dilemmas.

Suggested further reading

- Beauchamp TL, Childress JF. *Principles of Biomedical Ethics.* 4th edn. Oxford: Oxford University Press, 1994.
- Pellegrino ED, Thomas MA, David C. *For the Patient's Good: The Restoration of Beneficence in Health Care.* Oxford: Oxford University Press, 1989.

Determining your generic skill requirements from the 'Person Specification'

For training posts, those generic skills that are required should be explicitly stated in the interview pack that is sent on request. They are usually found under the heading 'Person Specification'

The table that follows is an adapted version of the 2007 Person Specification for entry to General Practice at ST1 level. It highlights some generic skill requirements:

	Essential selection criteria	How evaluated
Clinical skills	• Clinical knowledge and expertise Capacity to apply sound clinical knowledge and awareness to full investigation of problems	Application form Interview/Selection centre References
Personal skills	• Empathy and sensitivity Capacity and motivation to take in others' perspectives and to treat others with understanding • Communication skills Capacity to adjust behaviour and language as appropriate to the needs of differing situations • Conceptual thinking and problem solving Capacity to think beyond the obvious, with an analytical and flexible mind • Coping with pressure Capacity to recognise one's own limitations and develop appropriate coping mechanisms • Organisation and planning Capacity to organise information/time effectively in a planned manner • Managing others and team involvement Capacity to work effectively in partnership with others	Application form Interview/Selection centre References
Probity	• Professional integrity Capacity and motivation to take responsibility for own actions and demonstrate respect for all	Application form Interview/Selection centre References
Commitment to specialty	• Learning and personal development Capacity and motivation to learn from experience and constantly update skills/knowledge	Application form Interview/Selection centre References

You will note that there is an overlap with 'The duties of a doctor registered with the General Medical Council', particularly in relation to relationships with patients and professional integrity. However, there are additional criteria and competencies listed here, for example in relation to coping with pressure and managing others.

These generic skills can all be tested during the interview itself.

Person Specifications on the web

- GP recruitment: www.gprecruitment.org.uk
- Modernising Medical Careers: www.mmc.nhs.uk

6.3 Questions that test your understanding of generic skills

As with questions that test your knowledge and understanding, it may be helpful to develop definitions of your own using buzzwords and key phrases. You are more likely to stand out and impress interviewers by avoiding the regurgitation of textbook definitions read by all of the candidates prior to the interview. If it is possible and appropriate, you can personalise your answer by supplementing it with an example from your own clinical practice.

Here are example questions that test your knowledge of generic skills:

'What do you believe are the qualities of a good doctor?'
This question gives you a great opportunity to demonstrate your knowledge of 'The duties of a doctor registered with the General Medical Council' and your understanding of the core ethical principles we have outlined. You should also consider the following statement from the GMC entitled 'Good Doctors':

> Patients need good doctors. Good doctors make the care of their patients their first concern: they are competent, keep their knowledge and skills up to date, establish and maintain good relationships with patients and colleagues, are honest and trustworthy, and act with integrity.

It is best to structure your answer around a few subheadings, for example:
- Patient care
- Clinical skills
- Communication skills
- Integrity
- Empathy
- Teamwork
- Leadership skills
   An example answer could be something like this:

> 'A good doctor should make the care of patients their first concern, treating every patient politely and considerately, with empathy and sensitivity, respecting patients' dignity and privacy.

'A good doctor should be able to apply sound clinical knowledge and awareness to clinical problems and make clear, sound and proactive decisions, balancing risks and benefits. Their aim should be to do the greatest good to their patient. Doctors must avoid causing harm and strive to protect their patients from harm (principle of non-malfeasance).'

'A good doctor should listen to patients and engage them in an equal and open dialogue. Good communication skills are also important for doctors when interacting with colleagues in team, leadership or management roles.'

'It is also important that a doctor has professional integrity, is honest and trustworthy, and is able to take responsibility for their actions. Furthermore, they should be able to admit when mistakes are made.'

As you can see from this example, by choosing a few subheadings that you think are the most important qualities of a good doctor, it should be possible to construct a decent answer.

'What do you understand an empathic doctor to be?'
The key buzzwords/key phrases that relate to empathy include:
- Understanding another person's perspective
- Sensitivity
- Personal understanding
- Creating a safe and understanding atmosphere
- Checking that individual needs are satisfied.
  So an answer to this question might be:

  'Essentially, empathy is about trying to put yourself in a patient's shoes. It is about being sensitive and attentive, and acknowledging patient's needs, in a warm and caring manner. Empathy is also about creating a safe environment for patients, and checking that their needs are satisfied.'

  'I find it important in my own practice to build up trust with patients, and this may require several encounters with a patient over a period of time.'

'What are the hallmarks of good communication skills?'
To be able to answer this question you need to have an understanding of what constitutes good communication.

Communication skills

Doctors should have good active listening skills as well as the ability to convey messages in a clear and effective manner.

Listening

Good listening skills are linked to empathy and should result in better rapport with patients, thereby generating mutual trust and better working relationships. Good 'active' listening skills include:

- Using appropriate body language such as an open posture and maintaining good eye contact
- Showing warmth and being supportive and caring
- Knowing when to stay quiet

Conveying messages

A doctor should also be able to convey messages to junior and senior colleagues, as well as patients and relatives in an effective and clear manner. Doctors should be able to adapt their communication to their audience. When conveying messages, doctors should:

- Use clear and unambiguous language, avoiding the unnecessary use of jargon
- Use a variety of communication media in addition to the spoken word such as the written word, diagrams and posters
- Check the understanding of the audience, if necessary adapting their message

---

Perhaps you would like to construct your own answer to the following question?

'Why should doctors admit if they make mistakes?'

This is a question about *professional integrity*. Consider the following responses when you construct your answer:

- Involving colleagues can rectify the mistake more quickly
- A doctor who admits to making mistakes (and hence takes responsibility for their own actions) will be trusted more by colleagues
- By admitting a mistake at an early stage, the matter can be resolved more promptly, rather than causing potentially more serious problems in the future
- It is stated in 'The duties of a doctor registered with the General Medical Council' that you should 'act without delay if you have good reason to believe that you or a colleague may be putting patients at risk'

'What are the attributes of a good team player?'

Consider these key attributes of a good team player:

- Considerate and able to compromise
- A good communicator with good listening skills
- Punctual and reliable with deadlines
- Role orientated, i.e. understanding their role and the role of others within the group.

When answering this question remember the importance of using individual examples from your own practice when you have had to work as part of a multidisciplinary team.

'What are the attributes of a good leader?'

It is important to distinguish between what makes a good team player as opposed to the attributes that make a good leader.

The attributes of a good leader include being:

- Diplomatic
- Approachable
- Adaptive
- Decisive
- Organised
- Flexible
- Inspiring.

Perhaps you would be best to choose attributes that belong to you. It is likely that the follow-up question will relate to your own leadership skills, at which point you will have already thought of examples from your own practice.

6.4　Questions that ask for examples from your own practice

It is quite possible that you may be asked a question that requires you to give specific examples of events or practice. If you are unprepared, these can be quite unpleasant in an interview situation, particularly if no obvious response springs to mind.

Although you cannot prepare for every eventuality, some prior preparation will probably come in useful. It might save you from undue stress on the day and spare you a failed interview.

These types of questions come in two forms. A question might ask for a *general* example such as:

- 'How do you organise your workload?'
- 'How do you keep up to date with your specialist knowledge?'

Alternatively you may be asked to give a *specific* example. Such questions could include:

- 'Tell me about a time when a nurse disagreed with your management of a patient. What did you do?'
- 'Can you give us an example from your clinical practice where teamwork was important?'

Having a personal 'database' of examples demonstrating most of the generic skills is likely to serve you well if you get asked this type of question.

6.5 Common questions that ask for *general* examples from your own practice

'How do you keep up to date?'

This question is testing the statement in 'The duties of a doctor registered with the General Medical Council' that you must 'Provide a good standard of practice and care . . .' and 'keep your professional knowledge and skills up to date'.

To support your answer you could give examples of some of the following methods for keeping up to date:

- Problem-based learning (PBL)
- Teaching that you have given or received
- Attendance at a course
- How you have acquired continuing professional development (CPD) points
- Journals that you have read
- The online resources that you have used.

'What are your strategies for the recognition and management of stress?'

The 'capacity to recognise one's own limitations and develop appropriate coping mechanisms' is part of the essential selection criteria in the GP 'Person Specification'. It is important that doctors can tell the difference between being under pressure and performing well, and being under pressure when performance is affected. Doctors need to be able to:

- Recognise the signs of stress
- Recruit people to help
- Develop strategies to resolve stress, both short-term solutions, such as asking for help, and long-term strategies. Dr Pinkus from the House of God, goes 'running for fitness and fishing for calm' (Samuel Shem, *The House of God*, 1979)
- Reflect—this should be a continuous process.

> **Other questions that ask for more *general* examples**
>
> 'How do you deal with criticism?'
> 'How do you organise your workload?'
> 'How do you organise your own finances?'
> 'Tell us about your time management skills.'

6.6 Questions that require *specific* answers from your own practice

> **Tips on preparing answers to questions that ask you for specific examples**
>
> **1.** Think about the generic skills you are being asked to demonstrate.
> An interviewer will usually be asking this type of question in order for you to demonstrate some generic skills (or a particular generic skill). This may be obvious. For example, if you are asked '***Can you give an example where teamwork was important?***' then it is fairly obvious that you are being asked the question in order to ascertain your teamwork skills.
>
> With some questions, the generic skill requirement is less obvious. For example: '***Describe a time when a nurse disagreed with you about a patient's management***'. However, with a little thought, you might be able to demonstrate a number of important skills when answering this question, including:
> • Communication skills
> • Ability to work in a team
> • Ability to involve your seniors.
>
> **2.** Be specific
> This may seem obvious, but it can be tempting in an interview to describe how you would generally deal with a situation, for example, if you were asked '***Describe a time when a nurse disagreed with you about a patient's management***' you should not reply with 'When I find myself in a situation where a nurse doesn't agree with me I generally speak to my Consultant and the Ward Sister'. The interviewer is looking for a more specific answer, highlighting an example from your own experience.
>
> Giving well-structured answers with well-chosen examples that highlight a range of generic skills is the best way to impress the interviewers.
>
> **3.** Keep the clinical details to a minimum
> The focus of most of these questions is on testing your generic skills, rather than your clinical knowledge. You should avoid giving too much information about

Continued

Continued

the medical details of the case. Instead, talk about the issues that were involved, and how you went about solving them, what the outcome was and what you learnt.

4. Consider non-medical examples
Much of the time it is more appropriate to use a work-related experience to answer generic questions that require an example. However, there may be instances where a non-work-related example highlights the required skills better, particularly if you are a relatively junior doctor answering questions about administrative or management experience. If you have been involved in activities that utilise generic skills, such as organising meetings or events, it might be worth using these.

5. Avoid examples where things went terribly wrong
Try to provide examples with happy endings. Similarly, if you are asked *'Tell us about a time when you made a mistake'*, you should avoid examples where there was a catastrophic outcome for the patient.

6.7 The STAR technique

When preparing and delivering answers to questions asking for examples, you can use the well-recognised STAR technique to structure your answer. STAR stands for Situation, Task, Action, Result. This technique can also be referred to as the SAR technique when 'Situation' and 'Task' are combined.

How to structure your answer using the STAR technique

1. Situation
Describe the situation or 'set the stage'. Keep the detail to a minimum. The aim here is to set the scene for the rest of your answer.
2. Task
Identify the task performed.
3. Action
Describe:
- What you did
- How you did it
- Why you did it
4. Result
Complete the story by saying what the outcome was and, importantly, what you learnt from the experience.

The STAR technique is applicable for answering any question that asks for specific examples. You need to think of experiences you have encountered prior to the interview but don't be tempted to make things up. Interviewers may be able to distinguish lies through lack of detail, inconsistencies or vagueness of the answer.

When answering questions don't be tempted to use other people's examples. It will be wrong, unconvincing and you don't know how many other people might be using them too!

Here we demonstrate how you answer a generic skills question that asks for a specific example.

'Describe a time when your communication skills made a difference to the outcome of patient care'

Using the STAR technique, and bearing in mind the hallmarks of good communication skills, this question could be answered as follows:

1. Situation/task
   'I was working as a Foundation level 2 doctor on the Acute Stroke Unit. An 85-year old lady was admitted with dysphagia and left sided weakness. The team felt it appropriate to feed her via a nasogastric tube. The patient and her husband had concerns and declined this . . .'

2. Action
   '. . . As the ward doctor, I had developed a rapport with the patient and her family and was able to spend time with them to explain the advantages and disadvantages of this intervention. I listened to the fears and concerns of the patient and her husband and was able to reassure them . . .'

3. Result
   '. . . She then consented to naso-gastric feeding and was later transferred to the Stroke rehabilitation unit where she made a good recovery. The patient would not have made such good progress had she not been fed. I felt that I made the difference because I was able to spare the time to listen and explain the procedure to the patient. I learnt the importance of gaining patients' confidence and trust.'

You can see from this example that the bare minimum of clinical detail is given. The answer highlights empathy, good communication skills and sound clinical judgement.

'Describe an example when demonstrating empathy towards a patient proved to be helpful'

When thinking about examples from your experience, consider some of the following situations:

- Dealing with sensitive situations (telling an elderly patient that they shouldn't be driving)
- Breaking bad news
- Speaking to a recently bereaved relative
- Dealing with a patient worried about a chronic disease.

More generic skills questions that require *specific* examples

Here is a list of scenarios to think about when preparing for questions asking for specific examples.

'Can you think of an example when:'
Empathy
- ***'You needed to demonstrate empathy towards a patient?'***
- ***'You had to support a colleague with a work-related problem?'***

Communication skills
- ***'Your communication skills made a difference to the outcome of patient care?'***
- ***'A nurse disagreed with you about a patient's management?'***
- ***'You had to break bad news?'***
- ***'You had to deal with a sceptical patient or relative?'***

Conceptual thinking and problem solving
- ***'You had to use creative thinking to solve a problem at work?'***

Coping with pressure
- ***'You were involved in a stressful situation at work and how you dealt with it?'***
- ***'You had to deal with an angry patient?'***

Organisation and planning
- ***'You had to manage a budget?'***
- ***'You had to construct an on-call or clinic rota?'***

Managing others and team involvement
- ***'You had to negotiate with a colleague?'***
- ***'Teamworking was important?'***
- ***'You had a leadership role?'***

Integrity
- ***'You had to demonstrate professional integrity?'***
- ***'You made a mistake at work. What did you do?'***
- ***'You had to defend your beliefs with regard to the management of a patient?'***

Although this list may appear quite daunting at first, you should be able to think of a few experiences that cover a number of generic skills. For example, dealing with an angry patient allows you to demonstrate your communication skills, as well as how you coped under pressure.

With a few well-chosen and prepared examples you should be able to cover all of these likely questions. If you can manage this, you will be much more confident at interview.

6.8 Questions based upon a scenario

Interviewers may give you a scenario that incorporates a problem or ethical dilemma. You may then be asked to solve the problem or state how you would react to the situation. This is designed to test your understanding of the issues involved. It also indicates how you respond under pressure. You can be given a scenario using a patient simulation exercise or role-play that focuses upon your clinical skills. Examples of these are covered in the next chapter.

Scenarios that relate to ethical and legal aspects are common. It is not possible to give you a thorough overview of all of these issues in Medicine. We have summarised those that we feel are most important for you to know about in your preparation for interview.

Scenarios based around the doctor–patient relationship are the most likely scenarios that you will encounter, but you could also be faced with scenarios involving work colleagues. Some of the common themes are:

- Capacity and consent
- Confidentiality
- Breaking bad news
- Difficulties with work colleagues.

6.9 Capacity and consent

It is essential to have a basic understanding of the basic principles that relate to capacity and consent.

Issues that relate to capacity and consent

You should be satisfied that you have consent or other valid authority before you undertake any examination or investigation, provide treatment or involve patients in teaching or research. Usually this will involve providing information to patients in a way they can understand, before asking for their consent.

Continued

Continued

What is informed consent?

Informed consent is a legal condition whereby a person can be said to have given consent based upon an appreciation and understanding of the facts and implications of an action. The individual needs to be in possession of relevant facts and also their reasoning faculties.

Assessing competence

Doctors tend to talk about *competence* whereas the law uses the term *capacity*. In a legal context, capacity refers to a person's ability to perform specific acts such as making a will, or giving or refusing consent to medical treatment. Doctors might be asked to comment on, or formally assess, a patient's capacity (competence) to perform such acts.

A patient is considered to have capacity if they are able to:
- Understand the information relevant to the decision
- Retain that information
- Use or weigh that information as part of the process of making the decision
- Communicate their decision (whether by talking, using sign language or by other means)

Other key points

- *Capacity is 'function specific'*: it does not refer to global competence or incompetence. One can only talk of capacity to perform a particular task. Thus a patient may be competent to make a will but incompetent to consent to a particular operation (or vice versa)
- *An imprudent decision is not, by itself, sufficient grounds for incapacity*: a person should not be regarded as lacking capacity merely because they are making a decision which is unwise or against their best interests
- *The standard of proof is 'the balance of probabilities'*: the usual standard for proof in civil cases is 'balance of probabilities' — as opposed to 'beyond reasonable doubt'. Thus, in assessing capacity, courts will be concerned with whether the balance of probabilities favours capacity or lack of capacity.

Mentally incapacitated patients

No one can give or withhold consent to treatment on behalf of a mentally incapacitated patient. You must first assess the patient's capacity to make an informed decision about the treatment. If patients lack capacity to decide, provided they comply, you may carry out an investigation or treatment, which may include treatment for any mental disorder, that you judge to be in their best interests. However, if they do not comply, you may compulsorily treat them for any mental disorder only within the safeguards laid down by the Mental Health Act 1983, and any physical disorder arising from that mental disorder.

Continued

Continued

Advance statements

If you are treating a patient who has lost capacity to consent to or refuse treatment, for example through onset or progress of a mental disorder or other disability, you should try to find out whether the patient has previously indicated preferences in an advance statement ('advance directives' or 'living wills'). You must respect any refusal of treatment given when the patient was competent, provided the decision in the advance statement is clearly applicable to the present circumstances, and there is no reason to believe that the patient has changed his/her mind. Where an advance statement of this kind is not available, the patient's known wishes should be taken into account.

Fraser ruling competence (Gillick competence)

This refers to a case in 1985 when a child was requesting contraception against her mother's (Mrs Gillick) wishes. The Law Lords, led by Lord Fraser, ruled that children under the age of 16 can consent to treatments (medical, surgical, dental, which would include abortion) if they are capable of understanding the nature and possible consequences of the procedure.

No lower age limit was specified. They advised that children should be strongly advised to discuss treatments with their parents, but health professionals could not inform them without the child's consent.

Given that issues relating to competence are rarely clear-cut, it is worth noting a few points for the purposes of an interview.

It would be appropriate to state that where you are unsure about the consent issues for a specific scenario you would want to discuss the case with a senior colleague and, if still uncertain, with your medical defence union. Very occasionally, a court ruling is required.

'How would you go about obtaining informed consent from a patient who was in a vulnerable position?'

This question tests not just your ability to obtain informed consent, but also your communication skills. In particular, it tests your ability to adapt your communication to the appropriate situation.

Further reading

- *Seeking Patients' Consent: The Ethical Considerations* is a booklet available on the GMC website: www.gmc-uk.org

6.10 Confidentiality

The GMC states 'Patients have a right to expect that information about them will be held in confidence by their doctors. You must treat information about patients as confidential, including after a patient has died'.

There are, however, instances where confidentiality may be broken, for example when:

- *The patient gives implied consent.* For example, if you refer a patient to a colleague, or if a patient brings along a family member to a consultation and starts discussing their condition.
- *Where disclosure is required by law.* For example if information is requested by a court or required on a death certificate.
- *There is a need to protect patients.* For example, where a crime is involved, or a situation where you discovered that a colleague was HIV positive and performing invasive procedures.

The following tough questions explore some of the instances where confidential information might be disclosed without a patient's consent. If you find yourself able to answer these comfortably, then the interview should hold no fears for you.

'A 14-year-old girl asks you for a second termination of pregnancy. How do you handle the situation?'

To answer this question it is important to understand some important concepts:

- Persons under the age of 16 are owed the same duty of confidentiality as those over the age of 16 assuming that they are Fraser competent (see earlier).
- Are there exceptional circumstances where confidentiality could be broken?
  - A problem would arise if you considered that she lacked Fraser competence. If she asked you not to disclose information about her condition or treatment to a third party, you should try to persuade her to allow an appropriate person to be involved in the consultation. If she refused and you were convinced that it is essential, in her medical interests, you may disclose relevant information to an appropriate person or authority. In such cases you should tell the patient before disclosing any information.
  - If you believe that she may have been a victim of physical or sexual abuse and that she cannot give or withhold consent to disclosure, you must give information promptly to an appropriate responsible person or statutory agency, where you believe that the disclosure is in her best interests.

'A patient of yours suffers from a serious mental illness. He is often erratic and unstable. You know that he drives, although you have warned him that it is often unsafe for him to do so. He insists that his illness does not affect his judgement as a driver. Should you tell the DVLA?'

The DVLA is legally responsible for deciding if a person is medically unfit to drive. The Agency needs to know when driving licence holders have a condition which may now, or in the future, affect their safety as a driver.

Where patients have such conditions you should:

- Make sure that patients understand that the condition may impair their ability to drive. If a patient is incapable of understanding this advice, for example because of dementia, you should inform the DVLA immediately.
- Explain to patients that they have a legal duty to inform the DVLA about the condition.
- If necessary suggest that the patients seek a second opinion, but advise them not to drive until the second opinion has been obtained.
- If you do not manage to persuade patients to stop driving, or you are given or find evidence that a patient is continuing to drive contrary to advice, you should disclose relevant medical information immediately, in confidence, to the Medical Adviser at the DVLA.
- Before giving information to the DVLA you should try to inform the patient of your decision to do so. Once the DVLA has been informed, you should also write to the patient, to confirm that a disclosure has been made.

'A child in your practice has recently been taken to hospital suffering serious injuries from abuse. His father is now being prosecuted. You have been asked to provide information about the child and his family for a case review. You are the GP to the child's father and he won't give consent to the release of information, what should you do?'

Case reviews are often set up to identify why a child has been seriously harmed, to learn lessons from mistakes and to improve systems and services for children and their families.

Where the overall purpose of a review can reasonably be regarded as serving to protect other children from a risk of serious harm, you should co-operate with requests for information, even where the child's family does not consent, or if it is not practicable to ask for their consent.

'A patient of yours is a doctor, and you are concerned that he has a drinking problem which could affect his judgement. It has taken you a long time to get him to admit to any problems, and if you disclose the information to his employer or the GMC now he will probably deny everything and find another doctor. What should you do?'

This patient has the same right to good care and to confidentiality as other patients. But there are times when the safety of others must take precedence. If you are concerned that his problems mean that he is an immediate danger to his own patients, you must tell his employing authority or the GMC straight away. If you think the problem is currently under control, you must encourage him to seek help locally from counselling services set up for doctors or for the public generally. You must monitor his condition and ensure that if the position deteriorates you take immediate action to protect the patients in his care.

Further reading
- *Confidentiality: Protecting and Providing Information.* Available on the GMC website: www.gmc-uk.org

---

6.11 Breaking bad news

It is common to be asked at interview how you might break bad news to a patient, and it is a question that you should be prepared for.

'You are asked to inform a patient that they have lung cancer. How do you go about this?'

You should be able to use an example of where you were involved in breaking bad news. You should also be aware of several important principles when breaking bad news.

Considerations when breaking bad news

Make sure that you are prepared
- Be fully aware of the results and understand the implications and options for the patient.
- Be knowledgeable about the condition and if necessary read up, look at websites and speak to other professionals.

Continued

Continued

- Allow sufficient time for the consultation and make arrangements so that you don't get disturbed (e.g. tell the receptionist not to put calls through to you or get someone else to hold your bleep)
- Ask a nurse to sit in with you. Ask the patient to come accompanied if possible.

Breaking the news
- Ask questions to find out the patient's current level of understanding
- Explain what has happened so far. Gauge their reaction and adapt your speed accordingly. When you feel it is appropriate, explain the diagnosis and give the patient time to react.

Consider the holistic needs of the patient
- Physical: what is the next step for the patient, and what treatment options are available (surgical, medical or palliative)?
- Psychological: how are they reacting? What support do they already have (friends and family) and what additional support can be provided (support groups, Macmillan nurses)?
- Social: what implications are there for the patient's work, lifestyle and family? What additional help can be provided (e.g. social security benefits)?

Ending the consultation
- Summarise everything that has been discussed
- Give the patient any relevant leaflets and information to take away
- Make any appropriate referrals
- Arrange for a follow-up consultation.

6.12 Difficulties with work colleagues

'One of your colleagues arrives constantly late for work in the morning. What do you do?'

You have to be careful when answering this common question. It is likely that the interviewer is looking for an empathic response. It is essential that you explore the reasons that may be underlying this problem. You should then try to work with your colleague and assist him or her in finding solutions to any difficulties.

A likely follow-up question is that this person continues to exhibit the same behaviour, despite your comments and help.

At this stage it becomes reasonable to advise the individual that things have to change, and that you have to alert his behaviour to a more senior colleague if they do not.

Finally, as stated in 'The duties of a doctor registered with the General Medical Council', you should be prepared to 'act without delay if you have good reason to believe that a colleague may be putting patients at risk'.

'One of your partners at work is feeling low and asks you to prescribe him antidepressants. What do you do?'

This seems like a nasty question but actually it's a great opportunity for you to demonstrate empathy, professionalism and knowledge.

The GMC's guidance *Good Medical Practice (2006)* states:
- Avoid treating yourself and those close to you
- Independent medical care should be sought whenever you or someone with whom you have a close personal relationship requires prescription medicines.

Self-prescription and prescription for colleagues are discouraged, therefore your answer should be no. Be supportive and, if necessary, offer to cover for your colleague so that they can see their own doctor.

6.13 Summary

- Be familiar with the four ethical principles, 'The duties of a doctor registered with the General Medical Council' and the 'Person Specification' for the post that you are applying for
- Think of examples of your generic skills in advance of your interview
- Learn a basic knowledge of the important ethical and legal issues in health care.

Chapter 7 **Competency-based tasks**

7.1 Introduction

This chapter covers some of the additional methods used for selecting candidates. These may complement or replace the traditional medical interview format. The selection methods covered in this section include:
- Patient simulation exercises
- Prioritisation exercises/written exercises
- Group tasks
- Making a presentation
- Tests of medical ability.

Many of these methods are already commonly used for GP Vocational Training Scheme and ST selection. The precise details will vary significantly between Deaneries. The use of these selection methods is increasing, and may eventually replace the traditional structured interview.

It is essential that you are aware of your interview format in advance so that you can adequately prepare.

These alternative forms of assessment give you opportunities to parade your strengths and demonstrate your suitability for the post that you are applying for. Effective preparation will give you the edge over your competitors.

7.2 The patient simulation exercise and communication tasks

This selection method typically involves a simulated patient interaction in the context of a clinical scenario. The candidate usually assumes the role of the doctor and an actor takes the role of patient. You may be familiar with similar

How to Succeed at the Medical Interview By C. Smith and D. Meeking. 2008 by Blackwell Publishing, ISBN: 978-1-4051-6729-1.

assessments if you have sat postgraduate examinations such as the PACES component of the MRCP examination.

Candidates are usually given a briefing sheet to read 5 minutes before the simulation. This will give clinical information or a background to the case scenario.

Typical scenario examples include:
- Taking a clinical history from a patient
- Breaking bad news to a patient
- Explaining an investigation or diagnosis to a patient
- A scenario that deals with an ethical dilemma
- Dealing with an angry patient or relative(s).

What is being tested?

These exercises are used to test a variety of qualities. These are usually the skills that are outlined in the 'Person Specification' for the post. These are typically the generic skills described in the previous chapter. The important skills are:
- Empathy and sensitivity
- Communication skills
- Conceptual thinking and problem solving
- Knowing your limits.

There tends to be less emphasis on clinical knowledge in these exercises, so try to avoid too much clinical detail. You should attempt to deal with these scenarios as you would when encountering them in your professional role and avoid the temptation to 'act' or 'role-play'. To maximise your chances of success, it is useful to be aware of the scoring system being employed as part of the assessment.

How to score points

With these exercises, the majority of the points you score relate to your communication skills. You should also be able to demonstrate clinical knowledge, for example the construction of a sensible differential diagnosis list where appropriate.

A typical mark-sheet for a patient simulation exercise will be as follows. Note the emphasis on listening skills and clear communication:

Task	Score (0, 1, or 2)		
Builds rapport with the patient	0	1	2
Elicits patient ideas, prior knowledge, concerns, expectations, etc. (including psychosocial issues)	0	1	2

Task	Score (0, 1, or 2)		
Demonstrates confidence about the clinical situation	0	1	2
Explains issues in clear language, using appropriate sensitivity	0	1	2
Checks the patient's understanding	0	1	2
Total	10		

Here are some tips for patient simulation exercises:

Starting the exercise

- Build a rapport. Stand up, shake hands with the patient and invite them to take a seat. Ask them how they would like to be addressed, how they are feeling and then ask 'How can I help you today?'
- If the scenario involves breaking bad news, consider asking if anyone has come along with them, and would they like to join the conversation. Of course, there won't be anyone else waiting, but this looks thorough and impressive to interviewers.

During the exercise

- Use active listening skills with your patient, and never interrupt them
- Avoid excessive focus on the medical details
- Probe for why the exercise has been chosen
- Avoid jargon and use simple language
- Know your limits. If you are in doubt as to whether you can help, be honest, and say that you would ask a colleague or explain how you would refer to an appropriate specialist
- Ask, if appropriate, about the patient's ideas, concerns and expectations
- Try to be patient-centred by involving them in any decisions that are being made.

Towards the end of the exercise

- Ask the patient if they would like to summarise what has been covered. This is a good way of checking their understanding
- Arrange follow-up with the patient and provide a safety net. For example, 'if you haven't heard from the hospital within a month, or if you are not improving, I would like you to come back and see me'

How to prepare for patient simulation exercises

There is a wide range of patient simulation exercises that you may be given. Most of these should relate to experiences you have already encountered as a practising doctor.

Common examples include experience with stressful situations such as dealing with angry patients or breaking bad news.

Before your interview, try to take some time to reflect on these experiences, considering the aspects that went well, and those that didn't go so well. Consult medical friends or colleagues with experience of video consultations (until recently a common feature of training for General Practice). These individuals will give invaluable personalised advice for conducting the optimal consultation.

Consider the following examples and how you would deal with them. You should feel comfortable in dealing with all of the scenarios described. Some helpful tips are incorporated alongside the descriptions. Here are some examples of scenarios you can face at interview.

Example consultation	Tips
You have to explain a diagnosis of diabetes to someone who doesn't speak or understand English well	Make use of non-verbal communication (e.g. draw diagrams)
You are presented with an elderly patient with poor compliance to her medication	Probe for a possible underlying problem, for example is the patient depressed? If this appears to be the case, ask gently about suicide: 'Do you sometimes feel that life is not worth living?' 'Have you ever thought about ending it all?'
A patient with a chronic condition, for example rheumatoid arthritis or multiple sclerosis, finds a new 'wonder drug' on the internet and asks you whether she could be prescribed it	You need to explore their current problems. Are they compliant with their current medication? What are their expectations? Are they unhappy with current treatment? Be honest: 'a lot of therapies are advertised on the internet, but many haven't been tested and may be unsafe. These drugs often don't work'. If it is a medication with which you are unfamiliar you should tell them you will investigate and ask other colleagues for their opinion
You need to explain the diagnosis of diabetes to a patient who works as a lorry driver	Explain the condition in a simple manner, avoiding medical jargon. With this question you need to be aware of the impact on driving. Is this occupation threatened by the diagnosis? If you don't know, don't guess. Explain that you will consult with the DVLA and get back to them

Example consultation	Tips
Breaking bad news	See Chapter 6
You suspect non-accidental bruises in a toddler brought in by his parents	For obvious reasons you must not jump to conclusions but keep the safety of the child in mind. Tell the parents that you are concerned and wish to bring their child into hospital for some tests. Explain that you cannot be sure of the cause, and that 'there are many conditions which can lead to easy bruising'. It is important to contact the Paediatric team immediately and inform them of your concerns
In the out-patient clinic you see a patient with a suspicious looking gastric ulcer noted during endoscopy. He requires a second endoscopy in 2 weeks. He is also the main breadwinner for his family, and has organised a holiday for them in 2 weeks' time	This scenario requires a full exploration of the psychosocial situation through careful listening and gentle questioning. If the investigation is essential, it seems likely that you will have to inform the patient of the potential serious nature of the problem
An elderly patient has dense cataracts but does not want an operation. His daughter is angry at you for not insisting upon an operation. She makes an appointment with you to discuss the situation	You will need to ask whether the patient is happy for you to discuss his medical details with his daughter. You need to explain the nature of the operation, and that you need to respect the wishes of the patient, taking into account issues of capacity and informed consent

7.3 The prioritisation exercise

These forms of assessment are designed to test competencies that include:
- Personal, organisational and administrative skills, particularly that you are able to prioritise conflicting demands and delegate to others when necessary
- The ability to cope under pressure, particularly the ability to recognise your own limitations and share the burden with others.

Prioritisation tasks are usually in the form of a written exercise. These have been used by Deaneries for General Practice selection.

Typically with such an exercise, you will asked to imagine that you are working as either a GP or a junior doctor and are given a list of several tasks (typically about six) that need to be completed within a limited time period (about 20 minutes). You will be asked to list the tasks in order of importance/priority, then justify your chosen sequence with an explanation for each.

When completing such a task, you should remember that your explanations for the prioritisation are more important than the actual order that you generate. There is usually no one right or wrong answer.

Do not spend excessive time agonising over the precise order. It is not uncommon for candidates to run out of time before completing the exercise.

Usually the list of tasks you are given will include one that is of high clinical importance and one that is an issue that relates to your personal life.

Here is an example of a prioritisation task:

'You are a junior doctor working for a gastroenterology team on a Friday afternoon. The consultant ward round is due to start in an hour. How would you prioritise the following demands/tasks?'

1. You are contacted by security demanding that you move your car from in front of the mortuary before it is clamped
2. You get a text message from your partner who asks you to call him/her urgently
3. You are called by a GP asking for a discharge summary to be faxed across to his surgery because a 'recently discharged' patient has collapsed in his surgery
4. A nurse informs you that the relatives of a patient want to speak to you—the patient was given the wrong dose of medication overnight and is feeling a little dizzy
5. A nurse on a different ward asks you to see a newly confused patient who has been waiting 3 hours to see a doctor.

The following should be considerations when formulating your answer to this type of task:

- *Patient safety comes first.* Are there any emergencies where your quick intervention could make a significant difference to a patient's outcome? Situation 3 sounds like it could be, and it is not clear why the patient has collapsed in the GP surgery. It is conceivable that there is some important information contained in the discharge summary that might be of use to the GP
- *Delegation.* You will not be able to complete all of the tasks listed if you plan to start the consultant ward round in 1 hour. Sharing the workload appropriately with your colleagues is essential. For example, you could ask the ward clerk to fax the discharge summary to the GP, and ask a junior doctor colleague if they could review the patient who has become confused

---

Continued

Continued

- *Answer the question honestly.* When answering this question you may be tempted to leave phoning your partner or moving your car until last because you feel that your priorities should be with your work. Significant uncertainty and worries in your private life may cause you stress that can affect your ability to work. It would be reasonable to say that you would prioritise making a quick phone call to your partner to check that all is well
- *Show that you know your limits.* Do you feel comfortable speaking to relatives where there may be a complaint pending? This is likely to depend on the nature of the mistake and who was at fault. You may wish to get a bit more information about this from the nurse before deciding whether you can deal with this on your own, or whether it might be more appropriate to be dealt with by a more senior colleague at a later time
- *Show that you can think creatively.* Is there someone less busy who might feel happy to move your car?

7.4 Group tasks

Group tasks have been used by Deaneries for GP selection. They are often the least popular part of the selection process. Candidates frequently consider them to be irrelevant and difficult to prepare for. However, as with all components of the medical interview, understanding what the assessors are looking for and thinking in advance of an approach to the task will give you the best chance to succeed.

How do group tasks work?

Small groups of candidates are asked to work together to deal with a work-related scenario. Trained assessors are allocated to observe candidates during the group exercise and they assign ratings to candidates according to their communication skills and problem-solving ability. Typically the discussion will last 15–20 minutes.

One of the most common scenarios used is a role-play involving a problem with a work colleague. Typical scenarios could include a work colleague constantly arriving late, being lazy at work or being under the influence of alcohol. Each candidate is assigned a role, perhaps each being a junior member of the medical team.

With scenarios of this type there is often a hidden problem that requires exploration — for example, the work colleague in question is going through relationship difficulties at home.

Other types of group task could include:

- Planning a campaign, for example to improve vaccination uptake
- Planning to set up a new service, for example a Diabetes Clinic in a primary care setting
- A general discussion on a political or health topic such as efficiency in the NHS.

What is being tested?

Candidates are being tested on communication skills and problem-solving ability. Areas that assessors will focus upon include:
- Interaction
- Participation
- Teamwork
- Time keeping.

How to score points in group exercises

The assessors are principally looking for evidence of teamwork, effective communication and leadership skills.

Having sensible things to say and good ideas are a bonus, but not essential. You need to be sensitive and tactful, and avoid confrontation with other group members.

In advance of your assessment you should think about phrases that are helpful in ensuring that group tasks are successful. Here are some examples:

- When initiating the discussion:

  'This is an interesting scenario. It will require input from all of us. Has anyone had any experience with this sort of thing in the past?'

- You disagree with another group member:

  'I agree with what you say but . . .'

- Someone is drifting off the subject:

  'I'm getting a little lost . . . do you mind if we recap the main issues?'

- When nearing the end of the exercise:

  'We have efficiently covered the main topics. Does anyone else have any other points they would like to make?'

Example tasks	Tips
You are a group of junior doctors discussing four other medical colleagues	This might seem like an almost implausible situation but it is a real interview example.

Example tasks	Tips
with various problems. Doctor 1 is not performing at work, is missing clinics and is forgetting to hand in forms. Doctor 2 has made a number of clinical errors, but is generally considered to be a capable doctor. Doctor 3 is a promising surgeon, but arrogant and rude with nurses. He has no problems with his patients or fellow doctors. Doctor 4 is an asthmatic who has been stealing inhalers, having been informally warned before about not doing this. Discuss the issues	The key is to explore the reasons behind the individual doctor's actions with sensitivity and understanding. Help should be offered to problems, but also you as a group should be prepared to act without delay if you have good reason to believe that a colleague may be putting patients at risk
You and your GP colleagues want to set up a Primary Care Diabetes Clinic. Discuss the issues	When you are setting up a new service you need to consider the following: • *Planning*: have you identified a need? Do you have the resources? Do you need to make a business plan? • *Consultation*: have you consulted other stakeholders (e.g. Secondary Care Diabetes services, patient groups and managers)? • *Implementation*: what patients are you targeting? (Type 1 or Type 2?) How will you promote the service and educate staff? • *Audit*: is the service achieving its aims?
You and your GP colleagues are having a meeting to discuss how to improve the uptake of vaccinations	As well as discussing the reason why vaccine uptake might not be as good as hoped, you may wish to consider planning a campaign to increase vaccine uptake. With a campaign you should consider: • Who are you targeting? • What will be your strategy? • What are your educational aims? • Audit: is the campaign achieving its aims?
You are a group of junior doctors discussing how to tackle the high rates of *Clostridium difficile* on the ward	You need to understand the causes for the high rate of infection and institute a response to improve the situation
Your GP surgery has a budget of £25K to develop a new service, for example a smoking cessation campaign, a weight loss clinic, a family planning clinic or a	This type of question is designed to create different opinions. The key to remember here is that you come to a sensible decision based on rational discussion.

Example tasks	Tips
well woman clinic. Each group member is assigned one of these and has to prepare a small speech about why their service should be allocated the money. The group then discusses where the funding should go	Avoid being overly competitive. Remember that you are being assessed on how you integrate and interact with the other group members
You and your colleagues want to set up a practice website. Discuss how you will go about this	Points to consider include: • What content including clinical and non-clinical you wish to include • What budget you have • Who will be responsible for up-dating the site?

It is impossible to give a comprehensive list of all the group tasks you might have to perform. The above examples are a representative selection for you to ponder.

7.5 Making a presentation

Traditionally, being asked to make a presentation has been the domain of the Consultant interview. In recent times, however, they have become more commonplace at junior doctor interviews. Although the idea of presenting fills candidates with a sense of dread, they are an excellent opportunity to score points.

What is being tested when making a presentation?
Assessors are able to test a wide range of skills, the two most obvious are:
• The ability to articulate and communicate
• The ability to cope in a pressure situation.
  For junior medical posts, the topics that are frequently chosen are those that might normally be discussed. Here are some example topics that you might be asked to make a presentation on:
• Why have you chosen this specialty?
• What are the current issues affecting your chosen specialty at this moment in time?
• How do you see this specialty evolving over the next 10 years?
• Explain how you teach others
• Why are you the best candidate for this post?

Tips on presenting

Most of us will have sat through many presentations, and know that the standard is variable! It seems that the same common errors are repeated again and again. If you have never presented or have presented poorly in the past, it is worth spending some time preparing for this aspect of the interview.

The amount of time you will have to prepare will vary. If you have advance warning it is worth reading through presentation technique advice in more detail. There is a wealth of literature available. Candidates may be given advance warning prior to the interview, or they may have to prepare the presentation on the day of the interview. Some panels may expect you to have slides, whereas others won't. Either way, the content of your presentation, and the principle that you apply, should be the same. There is a brief summary below to aid you.

- *What are your main messages?* Determine what your main messages are before you even think of preparing your visual aids. The best presentations will convey three or four key messages. One of the main problems with presentations is that, despite good content, the messages are often lost in a mass of unimportant information. The messages must first be clear in your mind before you address your audience.

- *How are you going to structure your presentation?* Before you start to prepare your visual aids think about how you are going to structure your presentation. (A common mistake is to prepare a PowerPoint slideshow before the themes of the presentation.) You should be prepared to stand up and give your presentation without any visual aids. Remember you need to include an introduction, followed by an outline of what you are going to present, finishing with a summary.

- *Keep the visual aids simple.* Visual aids are there to augment the presentation but the main focus is you. Slides should summarise the main points but not be packed full of detail, nor should they be too flashy. Turning the slides off from time to time and talking directly to the audience is a powerful technique, and will keep the audience's attention.

- *Keep your prompts simple.* Effective presenters maintain eye contact with the audience as they speak, even if they are reading their presentation word for word. It doesn't matter if there are pauses whilst you read from your cues, but when you speak you should be directly addressing your audience. Keep your cues simple, but not too simple that you forget important content.

- *Practise!* Practise your presentation out loud as soon as you have prepared your first draft. Remember your messages need to be clear. You should also time your presentation. Bear in mind that many presentations run over time, which frequently frustrates interviewers and may lead to them being stopped early. Practise in front of an audience or video yourself if possible.

7.6 Tests of medical ability

Stations testing medical ability are a common feature at specialty-specific interviews for training posts. Medical ability can be tested either with a simulated patient encounter or by direct questioning by the interviewers.

What is being tested?

Stations that test medical ability are designed to assess a candidate's competence and ability to perform the job that they are applying for. Competencies tested could range from surgical skills to generic skills such as communication with patients and relatives. They also provide the assessors with clinical evidence of a candidate's commitment to that specialty. Tests of medical ability are likely to come in two forms:
- Tests of medical knowledge
- Tests of clinical skills.

How to prepare for the clinical skills station

- Firstly, it is important to be aware of the level of competency that is expected for the post for which you are applying. This information should be available on the relevant Royal College website
- Try obtaining feedback from other people who have been for similar interviews
- Make the most of feedback from assessments you may have received such as Direct Observation of Procedural Skills (DOPS) or from clinical examinations you have completed
- Try to ensure that you perform examinations and procedures correctly at work, so that you are able to be reproduce them naturally under stressful assessment conditions.

Example scenarios

Here are some examples of tasks that candidates have been given at interviews:

Specialty	Task
Medicine	ECG or chest X-ray interpretation Management of cardiac arrest Management of a tricyclic antidepressant overdose
Surgery	Discuss differential diagnoses, investigations and management of the acute abdomen Discuss the complications of hemi-arthroplasty Demonstrate incision and drainage of an abscess

Specialty	Task
Paediatrics	Simulated management of neonatal resuscitation
	Explaining a diagnosis of Type 1 diabetes to a child's parents
	Simulated management of a head injury in an infant
Ophthalmology	Fundus examination using a direct ophthalmoscope
	Use of microsurgical instruments to demonstrate suturing
	Assessment of stereoscopic and binocular vision
Psychiatry	Assessment of a man on a surgical ward who is confused and agitated
	Assessment of suicide risk after deliberate self-harm
	Discuss aspects of the Mental Health Act

7.7 Summary

Competency-based exercises at interview cause a lot of consternation for candidates. View them as an opportunity to shine more than other candidates. Give them some thought and prepare properly.

Finally, a few important principles:

- Find out as much information as you can about the interview format in advance to allow for effective preparation
- Practise assessment scenarios in advance of your interview
- Try to relax and behave naturally so that your own personality is easily revealed.

Final thoughts from an interviewer

Interviewing is very hard work. It has been made more so by laudable efforts to introduce a level playing field so that the same question is asked 30 times by panel members.

Although every effort is made to be fair, it is difficult not to let concentration drift as you listen for the 27th time to the definition of clinical governance being delivered in a flat monotone voice by an earnest, unsmiling candidate.

To maximise your interview chances, try to put yourself in the interviewer's shoes.

Without exception, the candidates I have interviewed who scored most highly are friendly, gently confident and show an interest in life outside of medicine. They have a self-deprecating sense of humour, smile a lot and engage every member of the panel when they speak.

Index